Statistics

for Health Care
Professionals

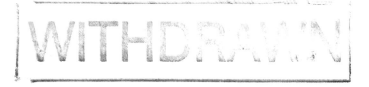

Statistics

for Health Care Professionals

An introduction

Ian Scott and Debbie Mazhindu

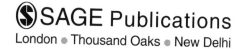

SAGE Publications
London ● Thousand Oaks ● New Delhi

SAGE Publications Ltd
1 Oliver's Yard
55 City Road
London EC1Y 1SP

SAGE Publications Inc.
2455 Teller Road
Thousand Oaks, California 91320

SAGE Publications India Pvt Ltd
B-42, Panchsheel Enclave
Post Box 4109
New Delhi 110 017

British Library Cataloguing in Publication data

A catalogue record for this book is available
from the British Library

ISBN 0 7619 7475 X
ISBN 0 7619 7476 8 (pbk)

Library of Congress Control Number available

Typeset by C&M Digitals (P) Ltd, Chennai, India
Printed and bound in Great Britain by Athenaeum Press, Gateshead

Contents

Statistics for Health Care Research

Areas of learning covered in this chapter

Who and what   is this book for?
How you can   use this book and use statistics to enhance practice
What is   evidence-based health care?
How are   statistics used to enhance evidence-based health care?
How statistics can help you to evaluate professional knowledge and
                professional values as the evidence base for practice (EBP).

Scope of the book

This book aims to expand health care students' and professionals' knowledge and understanding of statistics within health care practice. We hope that through reading and using this book you will be encouraged to evaluate statistical analysis and its relationship to evidence-based practice. There are many different approaches to investigating questions in health care practice. This book deals with quantitative approaches to investigating problems in health care, which require an understanding of some of the basic rules and principles of statistics. Understanding research in health care requires appreciating both qualitative and quantitative approaches to analysing data. Students of health care professions, both medical and non-medical, can expect to encounter a range of research approaches, which use particular statistical techniques to derive answers to particular patient problems. To this end, health care practice involves understanding of a range of research techniques within health-related subjects, including the use of statistics.

For many students and practitioners of health care, statistics is a subject that can often appear incomprehensible, daunting and, worse still, far removed from the real issues and problems encountered when caring for people. This book tries to demystify some of the more commonly used statistical tests and help readers understand the language of research that uses statistics, which both novice and advanced researchers find very off-putting to read. Undertaking the exercises within and at the end of each chapter will encourage you to think critically and reflectively about the research that you encounter, both in terms of the statistical process and the dynamic health care context in which studies are executed. This book can be used as a basis for taught courses on statistics at both pre-registration and post-registration level and as a reference guide for those using statistics in health care settings. The book is an introduction and aims to take you from novice to advanced beginner. Statistics is a vast subject which many people find difficult. We hope to make the learning process easier, but we can't promise an effort-free process.

> **Glossary**   When you see a term in **bold** you may want to look it up in the glossary of terms at the end of the book. This will explain terms used and help you to remember key words.

The book is divided into eighteen chapters. Each contains explanations of its terms and use for reference. A glossary has been provided and every time you encounter a word in **bold** print you can look up a short definition in the glossary. In the test at the end of each chapter you will find questions and exercises. Using these exercises will allow you to practise and become more proficient.

The book begins by taking a 'how to' approach, which explains how specific statistical tests can be performed. We have included details of how to calculate many of the statistics by hand. This is because doing at least some of the statistics by hand will help you to get a feel for the processes. As the statistical techniques become more advanced, readers are

> **Professional values**
>
> - To practice within the various codes of conduct, which regulate your chosen health care discipline.
> - Be aware of cause and effect of health and ill health.
> - Track progression and regression of health states and disease.
> - Serve society by implementing the best practice based on available evidence.
> - Teach new generations of health care Professionals by using up to date research findings.
> - To be self-governing and self-regulating in order to protect and serve the public.

directed towards suitable computer packages and other literature. This is because there are already excellent texts about some statistical concepts, which deal with some statistical techniques, although not many texts, have health care as a focus. This can make understanding statistics difficult for students of health care, as statistics often appear far removed from patient problems. Examples of statistical techniques commonly used will be explored and the results of a hypothetical questionnaire on sexual health and a clinical trial are used to encourage you to practise and explore statistics. We encourage you to try calculating statistics by hand, at least at first. This will help you to develop a feel for what is going on. Computers with statistical packages are not always available in health care settings. As tests become more advanced and you feel more confident, do use the statistical computer packages that are available. (A short guide to using SPSS and Excel can be found at www.sagepub.co.uk/resources/Scott)

Box 1.1

Reflective exercise

Take a few moments to think about the decisions made in health care today.

- How do we make decisions about what is the best care for patients and clients?
- How do you make decisions about what is best for you?
- How do you feel about making decisions that may affect another person's life?
- About people's health?
- About circumstances which may affect a person's ability to: give birth, father or mother children, recover from cancer, cope with devastating trauma, cope with loss or grief, help someone integrate back into society after mental illness

How do we as health care providers analyse such problems and then come to reach decisions that have an impact on many people's lives? The answers to these questions lies in the basis we use for our professional knowledge, the power we have to implement changes in practice and what constitutes our evidence base for our practice.

The use of clinical and community-based studies will form a central thread to allow data analysis to be explored from the perspective of differing subject areas. As well as analysing data from the studies provided we encourage you to analyse your own data, collected in response to some sample questions.

We encourage you to think critically about data analysis and research design and how appropriate research design impacts upon evidence-based practice. This is because an understanding of statistics is essential if the numerous reports and documents issued within the health industries are to be scrutinised and considered in a critical manner.

After reading the book, we hope that your skills of critical analysis will have become more refined. We hope that you will have a better understanding of the process of research and the use of statistics and all that is involved in getting answers to problems. We hope that you will be able to understand the importance of carefully reading and reviewing research reports in order to come to conclusions about their relevance to your area of practice. It is also hoped that you will begin to feel comfortable talking the language of quantitative research, which can assist you when presenting a case for changing or improving an area of practice.

The use of statistics in
health care research

There has been an increase in the development of research-based and evidence-based practice (EBP). For students undertaking professional health care education, and those practising as professionals in health care, understanding the statistical terms used in research is of paramount importance when evaluating research studies.

One of the key aims of this text is to enable the development of a greater understanding of the process and practice of using statistics in order to find answers to complex health problems.

After the initial preparation to practise health care, qualified practitioners are charged with a duty to care for patients and clients in the best manner possible. This means taking account of patients' and clients' family life and their involvement with others, the knowledge and skills attributed to practice, medical orders and the role of the allied health professions (AHPs). Understanding statistical terms helps practitioners to make sense of the many research studies that underpin EBP, takes account of professional values as service providers to the public and enables practitioners to undertake studies themselves.

What are the goals of health care research?

The primary goal of health care research is to aid patient and client care by developing a unique scientifically based body of knowledge which can be used to help us with decision making, to develop new practice and promote the professional role.

The degree to which a body of people such as health care professionals can be judged as professional resides to a large extent on the body of specialist knowledge that they can draw on for practice. Developing a specialist knowledge base by a process of scientific enquiry can aid the professional standing of a professional health care provider.

The ultimate aim of health care providers is the delivery of safe, effective care for patients and clients. This is an essential prerequisite in all health care professionals' codes of conduct.

Understanding statistics is just one way of ensuring that professional practice is based on the best available evidence to date by which to treat and help the wider community. Health care research shares many of the qualities of practice interventions, as they are both practical and intellectual activities, which have a defined language to learn. Good practice and good research do not spring from *ad hoc* or sloppy practice. Health care practice and health care research both use processes which when applied rigorously can improve patient care. Health care practice that is ritualised, not research-based and not assessed, not planned and (more important) not evaluated to see if it makes a difference to patient care can kill people, as it leads to unsafe practice. Evidence of this is to be found in the various catalogues of disciplinary hearings concerned with the safe conduct of health care providers of all disciplines.

Research, from whichever perspective, that is not rigorous, systematic, ethical and well designed can have devastating effects on people's lives. The thalidomide drug research is a case in point. Maynard (2003) suggested that medication errors occurring in health care in the United States kill twice the number of people who died in the terrorist attack on the World Trade Center on 11 September 2001. The prevalence of Methicillin-Resistant *Staphylococcus Aureus* (MRSA) in Britain causes great concern and many cases of atriogenesis. In France four times more antibiotics are consumed *per capita* than among Dutch patients, with higher levels of antibiotic resistance as a result (Maynard 2003). Understanding statistics in health care research, then, is every professional health care provider's business.

Professional knowledge and evidence-based practice

Florence Nightingale argued that systematic and routine data should be gathered from patient care settings in order to determine whether or not interventions were effective. Today implementing practice based upon statistical evidence is still problematic. The difficulties can to a large extent be attributed to the lack of engagement of health care providers in the process of change (Maynard 2003). Instituting change in health care relies on an understanding of statistics. Understanding the language of statistics gives all health care providers a common language despite the differences between the professions. The difficult question remains, however: in gaining consensus in deciding what exactly constitutes evidence? If we examine the credibility of evidence-based practice (EBP) in health care through exploration of its philosophical origins, there are several key features that emerge as important considerations. First, we need to evaluate critically the declared purposes and strengths of what exactly constitutes the evidence base for practice in health care. Second, we require an analysis of the implicit reasons for implementation of EBP. Third, we require a critical discussion of the strengths and limitations of EBP within the context of modern health care.

It is questionable whether evidence-based practice is a borrowed or unique concept. Whatever considerations and issues are raised, there can be no doubt about the impact of statistics upon the prevailing views of professional practice. The implications of ensuing debate on statistical concepts for health care providers are numerous and have significant implications for the future of the professions. This is because the implications range from immediate curriculum development and delivery of professional practice in health care education and training to a multi-professional and multicultural perspective, including the role and preparation of educators, clinicians and students. The **quantitative paradigm** has had a massive impact on the knowledge base for the practice of health care professionals. Some authors maintain that, philosophically, EBP is fundamentally utilitarian (Colyer and Kamath 1999). If that is the case, an understanding of statistics is essential for EBP.

Having read this chapter and completed the exercises, you should be familiar with the following ideas and concepts:

- Using this book to develop your understanding of statistics
- Evidence-based practice
- The relation between quantitative research and evidence-based practice
- How quantitative research contributes to the development of professional knowledge and professional values
- The importance of statistics in health care practice

Exercises

1   When considering introducing change to your practice, what type of evidence do you require to support that change?
2   Consider the last time change was introduced to your practice. What evidence was it based on? What role did you play in the decision? Did the change have a statistical basis?

2

The Statistical Approach:
When should it be Applied?

Areas of learning covered in this chapter

What are the major concepts in statistical analysis?
What types of studies use statistical analyses?
Where do statistics fit within the research framework?

In the first chapter we discussed how an understanding of statistics is essential if professionals are to engage with the development of professional knowledge and practice. But what are statistics? Why use the statistical approach and when should it be applied? How do we know if the right test has been used when reading and evaluating research?

What are statistics?

'Statistics' is a term that derives from the Latin *status*, meaning state, and historically statistics referred to the display of facts and figures relating to the demography of states or countries (Bhattacharyya and Johnson 1977). In French the term *recherche* (research) means to go and look for something. The statistical approach involves defining phenomena in terms of numbers and then using the numbers to either imply or deduce cause and effect. Statistics are a key research tool for quantitative researchers.

Box 2.1

Reviewing

Take a brief look at some quantitative studies. Make a note of the statistics used.

Today statistics are used in a whole variety of studies and investigations. Statistics are used to summarise and describe the data from studies where the data are collected in the form of numbers. Statistics are used to look for patterns and to ascertain the probability of observations having occurred by chance. Statistics are thus a vital tool that underpins all quantitative (number-based) research.

The scientific method

The process of collecting facts in a systematic manner is the basis of the concept of evidence-based practice. This is because, predominantly, knowledge for practice is predicated upon the belief that the world and its inhabitants can be viewed objectively, and predictions about things can be proved or disproved. Having a view about how knowledge is created and tested that is shared generally with other people in the world is called a 'world view' or **paradigm.**

Some beliefs associated with statistics from the quantitative and scientific paradigm:

- The quantitative approach, which has been termed the 'scientific method', is based on a number of beliefs. Scientists who have been influenced by the philosophical writings of Thomas Hobbes (1588–1679) and John Locke (1632–1704) traditionally used this method, derived from the school of thought known as logical positivism, which is associated with the beliefs of the French philosopher Auguste Comte (1798–1857). Comte held that human intellectual development could be characterised through three key stages: theoretical, metaphysical and positivist.

- Logical positivism is also based on the eighteenth century philosophical understanding of Hume (1888), which advocated that
  knowledge can be acquired through the careful observation of
  things and of people, their environments, customs, behaviours, and
  by observing physical matter, e.g. chemicals and other substances,
  to see how they behave (Kerlinger 1986). Logical positivists were
  suspicious of things that could not lend themselves to be observed
  or heard, like feelings and emotions (Burns 2000).
- Experiments use observation of things to determine effect of something upon something else in a controlled environment. This means
  that all factors that could affect the outcomes of a research are
  controlled or accounted for. A control group, to which nothing has
  been 'done', is needed and observations are then made of the
  behaviour of an experimental group, to which something has been
  done. Observations are made of both groups, and then compared
  and results deduced (which is why it is often called the deductive
  approach).
- Observations can then be ranked, coded, organised and analysed – in
  other words reduced to their smallest mathematical units – making it
  possible to predict outcomes of data, which can then be analysed
  mathematically (Russell 1919).
- One of the major doctrines of logical positivism is that numbers are
  the best basis for analysing research data as they remain untainted
  by feelings or emotions (Depoy and Gitlin 1993).
- Individuals are observers of the physical world set on discovering
  laws that, through careful theory testing and checking, can be
  used to govern the world and its inhabitants (Popper 1957).
- The laws governing the physical world can be represented as
  universal laws, which when applied can be used to predict outcomes
  by a process of hypothesising, testing, confirming or refuting
  (Popper 1963) and used to control the environment, e.g. the laws
  of thermodynamics.
- Individuals respond mechanically to their environment by obeying
  predetermined universal rules, e.g. touching a hot plate will produce
  the same reaction in individuals across the world (see also Brandt
  1928).
- This means that logical positivists believe that reality is not something known intrinsically by each individual but is something that
  lies outside the realms of individual perception and can be observed,
  counted, ranked, ordered and analysed objectively (Hume 1888,
  Locke 1975).
- A major belief of logical positivists is that events in the world all have
  causes, which can be discovered through the process of hypothesising and theory testing (Popper 1957, 1963, 1990).

Box 2.2

Where do you stand?

Take time to reflect on the ten points on the list. Which do you agree with? Are they interconnected? Can you logically agree with some but not all of them?

Given that quantitative studies tend to have a universal philosophy, they also tend to follow a universal method. This method is commonly known as the scientific method, although it is worth noting that the idea of the scientific method is not confined to quantitative research.

The characteristics of research methods that use statistics

These methods have a number of distinct qualities, although not all of these will be seen in every study. Studies based on statistics will generally attempt to control the influence of factors (variables) that are not important to the actual study but could bias the results. All statistical studies rely on evidence derived from observation or experiment as the basis of any new knowledge generated; such information is given the term 'empirical'. An important aspect of empirical evidence is that it is itself verifiable or provable by observation, experiment and or replication.

The majority of studies using statistical methods seek to test a hypothesis (an idea or theory); by 'test' we mean to disprove (*sensu*, Popper 1959). Thus studies based on statistics tend to involve the collection of empirical evidence in order to disprove a hypothesis. In general, when we use statistics, we try to produce results that are generalisable, that is, the results from a sample are applicable to the overall population of individuals we are interested in. The link between the sample and the population is the focus of many statistical tests.

Within research the statistical approach is used to:

- Describe variables and their relationships.
- Help explore the nature of relationships among variables.
- Help explore the differences between samples and populations.
- Help investigate the role of chance in giving rise to measurements.
- Help explain relationships between sets of data.
- Predict the causes of relationships among phenomena.
- Control for (take account of) variables.

Box 2.3

Using studies

Ram Patel works as a nurse in a neurological out-patient department. He is concerned that the level of immediate post-consultation care may be inadequate, particularly in view of the fact that many patients receive disturbing prognoses following their consultations. He decides to embark on a study to assess the impact of the consultation on his patients' immediate health. He intends to use the results to help make a case to increase the allocation of staff to post-consultation care. Ram is aware that he needs to take measures pre- and post-consultation.

- Should Ram take qualitative or quantitative measures?
- What quantitative aspects of health could Ram measure?
- What qualitative aspects of health could Ram measure?
- How could Ram use his data as part of an argument to justify more resources?

Do you think health care managers receive quantitative or qualitative data better? Why?

When we examine or establish research using statistics it should, more or less, follow the form described below. As it is not the purpose of this book to detail all the research methods, we will not go into detail of the different aspects of all the methods but focus on indicating where within the research approach adopted statistical analysis lies.

Basic parts of the research method

Forming the question(s)

Identify the problem or phenomenon of interest. Decide on the outline of the study, the population to be studied and the questions that will be investigated. Through searching the literature and drawing on your own thoughts decide on which methods will be used to gather data. At this stage a small pilot study may be conducted that will allow potential problems to be highlighted and obviously if any do come to light there will be a need to revisit the questions being addressed.

The literature review

There is a vast body of literature concerning many areas of health care; it is essential for any new work to be set in the context of any previous or concurrent work. It is also essential that the literature is reviewed such that we can learn from this work before we move on. The literature review will probably start from the moment a research idea is conceived; it will continue throughout the study.

Conceptual and theoretical frameworks

There are different ways of viewing problems. Many areas of investigation have distinct frameworks and concepts on which the evolution of new knowledge is based. It is important to be aware of these, for the particular type of study you are working on. It is likely that a biologist and a sociologist will use different concepts and attach varying levels of importance to different types of data. Despite having different lenses through which to view the world both these academic disciplines use statistics a great deal.

Hypotheses and variables

In many studies there is a hypothesis, a prediction or series of predictions that are under test. Normally the hypothesis will have originated from a theory. We test hypotheses by measuring relevant variables and investigating how they relate to each other and the populations from which they originate. A variable is a phenomenon (thing) that varies.

The research design

The design provides guidelines with which you conduct the research. The design directs the sampling technique, and how the data are to be collected and analysed. The principal aim of the research design is to minimise all the potential sources of error. It should also strive to ensure that any hypotheses that are under test are actually tested, i.e. the research design should allow the aims of the research to be met. At this stage you must also consider the ethical implications of your work.

Population and sample

The population is composed of all those individuals or objects that you could potentially take measurements from. The sample represents those individuals or objects (given the constraints and resources) that you were able to measure from. Normally we plan to take a sample that is representative of the population being studied. This is subject to the research design being approved by an appropriate ethics committee.

Data collection

You collect the data, using the method or tool most appropriate.

Data analysis

Here the data are described and summarised, and statistical tests are performed. There are many computer-based statistical packages available to help.

Results and conclusions

Having analysed the data, you need to decide what the results are suggesting. You need to decide whether or not any hypothesis under test has been confirmed or rejected. The results need to be related to those from previous studies, and the work needs to be related to an existing body of theory. You should also consider whether you have an ethical duty to communicate the findings of the study.

How do we know if the statistical analysis is any good? Analysing statistics critically

The major concepts involved and the statistical language become more comprehensible as you go on to practise and undertake the exercises at the end of each chapter.

As you become more familiar with statistics you will be in a position to make up your own mind whether you feel a research report that uses statistical analyses is of value. The process to use in making up your mind is the process of getting critical. Getting critical takes a long time, lots of practice and much reading of research reports. Do not worry if this seems insurmountable at this stage. Getting critical requires practice and an understanding of statistical concepts.

The process of becoming critical is ongoing and developmental. Once you have tackled an analysis of a research report, your skills will develop and refine. Reading from a wide variety of sources enhances the development of skills for becoming critical. Health care professionals should be encouraged to carry out and critically evaluate research in order to secure the best evidence base for care.

As you go through this book, and work through the exercises, we hope you will become more critical of how you view statistics. That is to say, we hope you will view all the statistics you are presented with with a healthy degree of suspicion and that your skills and knowledge (enhanced and honed through using this book) will enable you to evaluate whether the statistics have been applied appropriately and correctly.

A critical analysis should be a considered, balanced evaluation, that is, you need to be aware that a practice/theory gap exists even in the field of statistical analysis, which means that sometimes we need to make compromises.

Before starting an evaluation you will need to remind yourself of the steps in the research process and refer to the appropriate chapters in this book. A very important point to remember when carrying out an evaluation is that just because research is published it does not guarantee that the results of an investigation are either valid or reliable.

In Appendix 1 we present a framework that can help you evaluate the statistical components of research and other reports. Do bear in mind that there may be other aspects of the research, as well as the statistics that you want to focus on. When evaluating statistical aspects of research reflect on why statistics are used (see above). You can use Appendix 1 to help you practise to become critical. We suggest that you start using Appendix 1 once you feel you have become more familiar and content with the basic concepts of statistical analysis.

Having read this chapter and completed the exercises, you should be familiar with the following ideas and words:

- Statistics
- The 'beliefs' of quantitative research
- The research method
- The components of the statistical approach
- The basis of a critical approach to statistics

Exercise

1 Select three research papers that report quantitative research.

   (a) Identify where the steps in the scientific method lie within the paper.
   (b) Decide if the papers follow the 'beliefs' outlined in the list of beliefs
        as described in this chapter.
   (c) At this stage, how do you feel about the conclusions that the authors
        reach and the implications for practice?
   (d) What would you require before implementing a change?

Measuring, Sampling and Error

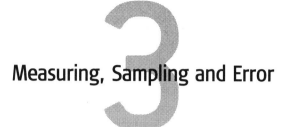

Whilst this book isn't about research design it's impossible to learn about statistics without knowing at least something about samples and populations. This chapter will take a look at the concept of the sample and the population.

Population

A population is made up of all the individuals or objects or phenomena that you could potentially measure/count as part of your study. If, for example, you were studying the reasons why nurses in the United Kingdom left the profession early, your population would be made up of all the nurses in the UK who had left the profession early.

If on the other hand you were studying the reasons why nurses in a particular hospital left the profession early, your population would be those nurses who left early in that particular hospital.

It is also important to note that the population that we are interested in may not be exactly the same as the one we end up sampling from. This is because some of the individuals in the population of interest may refuse to take part in our study. Thus there may be a distinction between the target population and the actual population.

Sample

In most cases it is unlikely that you would be able to gather information from all the population: you probably would not have the resources. So instead we must take a sample. A sample is made up of a proportion of individuals or objects from the total population. Many of the statistics described in this book concern establishing how good the sample is at representing the population and whether or not different samples come from the same population.

There is a great deal of literature concerned with how to ensure that a sample is representative. However, as this book is primarily about statistics we will not discuss them here, but we strongly advise you to read around this topic before embarking on any research. A useful chapter to read is chapter 6 of Blakie (2003).

Cases

Every sample is made up of the individuals or objects under study. These individuals or objects may be referred to by a variety of names, such as sampling units. For each individual or object we will measure some variable or variables. These variables may be physical (e.g. blood pressure), they may represent thoughts or feelings (e.g. anxiety) or represent events in the individual's life (e.g. number of visits to a health clinic). The important thing about these variables is that they are measurable. If a variable isn't measurable it can't be dealt with statistically. Each individual or object from which we take a measurement is termed a **case**.

Box 3.1

Measurements and samples

Go to a library and select five articles. For each decide on:

- The measurement.
- The variable being measured.
- The population.
- The sample.
- The sampling unit.

For each case the measurement may be referred to as a value. A collection of values is called data.

For every case we should be able to state: the measurement, the variable being measured, the sampling unit, the actual sample and the population being studied.

For example, say we were studying hypertension in populations living near ironworks. Our **measurement** would be 80 mm Hg, the **variable** would be diastolic blood pressure, the **sampling unit** would be individuals who are in the vicinity of the ironworks, the **sample** would be made up of those individuals from whom measurements were taken. The actual **population** is thus defined as all individuals willing and able to be measured living within the vicinity of the ironworks. (Note that the exact meaning of 'vicinity' would be determined by the researcher.)

Statistical and real population

In the example above there is a slight difference between population defined and the one that we originally intended to work on. The defined population includes the term 'willing and able' – obviously you can't take measurements from those not willing to take part in your study. Thus there can be a difference from the population from whom the measurements were sampled, often called the *statistical* population, and the real population or *biological* population, i.e. all those in the vicinity of the ironworks. So beware: not all individuals in a population are available to become sampling units. In some instances, what constitutes the

Table 3.1   A range of different variables and their likely sampling units

Variable	Sample	Sampling unit
Occurrences of MRSA on a ward	Wards which record occurrences of MRSA that you collected data from	Ward
Length of stay in hospital	Hospitals that record length of stay that you collected data from	Hospital
Pulse rate	Individuals that you record pulse rate from	Individual
Gender	Individuals whose gender you recorded	Individual
Hospital position in league table	Hospitals used to formulate league table	Hospital
Number of live births	Units of area from which records of live births have been collected	Unit of area

sampling unit and the variables being measured is not at first obvious. Look at the example in Table 3.1.

As you can see, the range of variables you can use is quite wide. You will also notice that some variables can be expressed as numbers on a scale, whilst others, such as gender, are discrete. This distinction is very important. Before you can identify an appropriate statistical test you must identify the type of variable and on which type of scale it is measured.

Measurement scales

Variables can be measured on a number of different scales. Three main types can be recognised: (1) nominal, (2) ordinal and (3) interval/ratio scales. These will now be discussed further.

The nominal scale

The nominal scale is the lowest on the scale hierarchy. Statisticians refer to a *hierarchy* of scales, because each scale further up the order contains the features of those previous. As the name implies, the data occur in named groups. Data are classified into the groups. The groups are mutually exclusive; an item of data can't be in more than one group. A good example of a nominal variable would be 'ethnic group' or 'home town'.

Ordinal scale

Ordinal scale data are similar to nominal scale except that the names of the groups contain an idea of rank or position. A good example here are the grades of staff nurses within a health service. The names of the groups, say 'staff nurse', 'charge nurse' and 'matron' convey an order or rank. The rank, however, does not suggest how much higher or lower the ranks are. The scale is used to arrange the measures from lowest to highest, but we wouldn't say that a charge nurse is twice as high as a staff nurse. Ordinal scales can be expressed in terms of names, as in the example here; as numbers, e.g. first and second in a race; and as letters, as in the UK system for grading nurses, e.g. A-I.

Box 3.2

For each of the variables in Table 3.1 state which scale you think the measurement would be made on.

Ratio/interval scales

In these scales ranks are used but this time the distance between the ranks is known and the distance between the scales is known. The points between the ranks can be subdivided. Ratio scales are similar to interval scales except that they have a true zero point. If, say, you recorded temperature you would know that the difference between 37°C and 38°C is 1°C. Thus the scale is interval, but the centigrade scale does not have a true zero point, thus it is not possible to say that 10°C is twice as hot as 5°C. An example of a ratio scale is weight; weight does have a true zero. Many measures of biological phenomena are measured on either the ratio or the interval scale.

Box 3.3

For the articles you selected in Box 3.1 now decide which measurement scales they have used. Remember, a study may use more than one measurement scale.

You should practise identifying appropriate scales. When we look at each statistical test, it is important to remember that it is the scale that the measurement is made on which largely determines the type of statistical test that can be applied.

Errors

Although in this book we do not largely concern ourselves with research design, it is important to think about how errors get into our study.

Indeed, a number of statistics that we shall discuss are really about taking error into account. When you conduct a study, error can occur in a number of different ways. Statistics can be used to account for or assess some of this error but not all. We will look at three types of error that you need to think about when conducting your own research or thinking critically about other people's studies. All studies have errors associated with them. The more error that is present the less you can rely on the study.

Measurement error

Measurement error occurs when we try to measure things. This is because most of the tools we need to use to measure things with are not 100 per cent accurate. Even if we are considering something as simple as recording the number of patients who turn up at a GP surgery, or taking a measurement with a ruler, measurement errors will occur. To some extent error associated with using instruments and apparatus to measure phenomena is easier to consider than error associated with methods, such as observation used to record human behaviours.

Box 3.4

Measurement error

Try measuring the length of the index finger from a sample of ten individuals. First use a ruler marked off in centimetres, then use a ruler marked off in millimetres.

Which set of measures shows the greatest variation (number of different values)?

What does this tell you about how useful the different rulers were?

Consider, for example, measuring the length of index fingers with a ruler that is divided into a centimetre scale only. When taking the measurement it would be difficult to record a measurement with a greater accuracy than 0.5 cm. A finger that was 5.75 cm long might be recorded as either 5.5 cm long or 6.0 cm long, and thus the study would have a measurement error. We could instead use a ruler with a scale that included millimetres. This would give a more accurate measure, but do note there is still error. For a finger that is 5.75 cm long (575 mm) we still need to judge whether it is 575 mm or 576 mm long, so we still have an error, albeit a much smaller one. Some people will say that the measurement is 575 mm and others 576 mm. This type of error is measurement error.

Measurement errors occur in most studies even when the variable is simply a count of something. The counters often make errors.

Measurement errors may be **systematic** or **random.** A random error occurs by chance and there is an equal chance that it will be either higher or lower than the 'true' value. Random measurement errors are not important if they are sufficiently small. A sufficiently small measurement error is one that is considerably smaller than the overall variation in the data. Systematic errors, on the other hand, are those that are consistently either smaller or higher than the 'true' value. Factors likely to lead to systematic errors need to be considered at the design stage.

To deal with measurement error you need to be aware of it. You should then choose a measurement tool that gives you the greatest level of accuracy, although you will need to consider the resources available to you. For example, high accuracy may involve spending more money or time. If you are using surveyors or interviewers make sure that you train them to use the data collection tools, e.g. the questionnaire.

Consistency

You also need to be aware that some errors will occur because measurement tools are not consistent. That is, for an individual item under measurement an instrument (e.g. a peak flow meter) will not always consistently produce the same measurement. Instruments need to be calibrated (measured against a known standard) before they are used. You then need to measure how consistent your instruments are between measurements, and between the individuals using the instruments. Then you can be aware of the error when discussing your results.

Box 3.5

Are your friends consistent?

Measure out five lengths of string. Each should be a different length. Now stand about 5–10 m away from a friend and ask them to guess the length of each of the bits of string. Show your friend one bit of string at a time. Now repeat until you have data from between five and ten of your friends.

Now look at your results, do some of your friends always overestimate or underestimate the length of the string? What type of error is that?

Do some of your friends seem to overestimate and underestimate in roughly equal proportions? What type of error is that?

Associated with consistency of instruments is consistency of the humans involved in taking measurements. This is known commonly as *inter-rater* reliability.

As we all know, humans are fallible. As such, where we are involved in recording measurements we are likely to make errors and be inconsistent. Take as an example the recording of accidents in factories. Some individuals report all accidents, however minor, whilst others will only record very serious accidents. Hence if you were conducting a study on reported accidents this inconsistency would introduce error into your study. When counting things, we are inconsistent. What is more, some people are more consistent than others. Thus elements of consistency must be considered in any study at the design stage. If you are using several individuals to collect data you must look at each individual to see if they are consistent with respect to themselves and with respect to other researchers. Consistency of measurement can be considered as a phenomenon both of measurement and of design.

Design error

Design error occurs, as the name implies, because the design of the experiment is flawed. There are of course varying degrees to which a study can be flawed and most studies are flawed in some way. If the design error is large, however, the study will need to be abandoned. This is why it is so important to get the design right. This book is not about research design methods but about statistical analysis. It is important to be aware of some of the errors you are likely to come across.

The most common error is that the sample is not drawn truly randomly from the population. Thus the conclusions drawn are not appropriate for the population as a whole. Often, particularly within research related to nursing, studies are based on single sites. This makes it difficult to draw general conclusions, as unfortunately the authors of such research often do. For example, a study of the performance of nurses in a particular hospital is likely to be biased by that hospital's working environment. It is unlikely that the results will be generalisable either nationally or globally.

The second most common error is to fail to take into account **extraneous variables**. Extraneous variables are those variables that, although not of interest, may alter the value of the variable being measured (often called the **dependent variable**). You may be able to control (hold constant) some of these extraneous variables. Time of day, light level, temperature, health status of participants, sex of participants, age of participants are all examples of variables that could influence the results of various studies. With careful design these variables can be eliminated as sources of error.

Box 3.6

For each of the articles you used for the exercise in Box 3.1 suggest what:

- Measurement errors have been made
- Design errors have been made

For each article reflect on whether they have discussed these errors and how they impact on the conclusions.

Besides controlling for the extraneous variables another important technique is to measure the extraneous variable and take into account its influence on the variable of interest statistically. To use this technique advanced statistical tests need to be used, and these are beyond the scope of this book. One problem researchers cannot account for is those extraneous variables that they may not be aware of before the start of the study. This is a surprisingly common problem. Although such problems can often be overcome, the best solution is a thorough reading of the research literature and careful design. Even then the problem can still arise; it's one of the joys of research.

Sampling error

Sampling error is the error that many statistical techniques try to take account of. Sampling error is the difference between the sample and the population. If we take a sample it is unlikely that the measure taken from the individual of the sample will exactly match that of the population. When we look to see how representative a sample is of the population or whether or not two samples come from the same population we need to take account of sampling error. Sampling error will increase the more variation there is among the sample you are measuring, and will decrease as the sample size increases.

The relationship between sample size, sample variation and sample error is important because one question you are bound to ask is 'How large should my sample be?' The answer is, it depends on the variation within the sample.

If you were working with the variable 'height', using a population of basketball players, the variation in height of this population would be very small, and thus the sample size that you would require would be small. If, however, you are working on variable height across the global population the variation would be large and a larger sample would be required.

Having read this chapter and completed the exercises, you should be familiar with the following ideas and concepts:

- Populations
- Samples and sampling
- Scales of measurement
- Consistency
- Measurement error
- Design error
- Sampling error

Exercises

1 For each of the studies below, indicate (a) the variable being measured, (b) the sampling unit, (c) the sample, (d) the statistical population:

   (i) A study on the impact of exercise on the bone density of women aged thirty-five to forty-five.
   (ii) A study on the different rates of outbreak of meningitis in villages in the south-west of England.

2 For the study on sexual health presented in Chapter 5 describe (a) the population and (b) the sample.
3 For the study on sexual health presented in Chapter 5 identify for four of the variables (a) the scale it is measured on (b) the measurement error that could be associated with it.
4 Summarise what you understand by the term 'sampling error'.

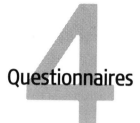

Questionnaires

Background to questionnaires

We have included a chapter on questionnaires because we recognise that many health-related studies have adopted this approach. However, the subject of questionnaires and research design is huge and cannot be addressed in detail in one chapter of a text this size. We aim to provide an overview and highlight some of the important considerations. A useful textbook about questionnaires is Oppenheim (1992).

Questionnaires can be used to provide additional information from people on a particular topic. The questionnaire described below uses closed questions, that is, the range of answers available was determined by the researcher. This type of questionnaire lends itself to statistical analysis.

Box 4.1

Questionnaire design

Two of the main questions to ask when thinking about designing a questionnaire are:

- What is it that I wish to find out?
- Is it to do with knowledge or attitudes or levels of understanding, or is it about behaviour or activities or decision making?

If you were going undertake a questionnaire-based study, what would you want to investigate?

The term **questionnaire** usually means a form containing a set of predetermined questions used for gathering information (**data**) from and about people as part of a **survey**. The term 'survey' is used to describe a research approach that attempts to cover as wide a range of the population as possible in order to obtain information about a subject.

Questionnaires can be used in various types of research, e.g. descriptive, comparative and attitudinal. There are many différent types of questionnaire. The type of questionnaire used will depend on the research question being asked. Questionnaires can be used to produce both qualitative and quantitative data. They can be used as a means to describe a population, to investigate cause and effect (Chapter 8) and to monitor change over time. Often questionnaires attempt to describe a population's behaviour, its attitude, view with regard to a certain topic, understanding of an issue or level of understanding. Surveys often use questionnaires in order to obtain such information. Sometimes an interviewer may also be used. People taking part in the survey are often termed *respondents, participants* or *subjects*.

A very helpful and informative textbook that discusses the background and detail of the main types of questionnaires can be found in Burns (2000). See also Oppenheim (1992).

When used as a quantitative tool, questionnaires help to put numerical indicators on these phenomena. As a quantitative tool questionnaires are a good method of collecting data, although such data can tend to be superficial, as there is no room for probing or extracting the meaning of the responses.

Questionnaires are a cost-efficient way of collecting large quantities of data in a short space of time, and if the questionnaire is properly structured large quantities of data can collected and subjected to statistical analysis. Once a questionnaire is constructed, it is usually referred to as an instrument or tool. The methods by which questionnaires can be administered include not only face-to-face interview but also telephone, mail, e-mail and World Wide Web.

Sample questionnaire

In Box 4.2 we describe a questionnaire that describes the behaviour of a group of people. (Please note that the full questionnaire is given in Chapter 5.) Let us say, for example, you wanted to know more about the epidemiology of AIDS and HIV in the United Kingdom. It might be useful to know more about the general sexual health of the population in the United Kingdom.

Safe sex is much discussed in the media, and one way of keeping safe is to use barrier methods of contraception. Large amounts of money are spent by governments on health promotion programmes to educate the general population about safe sex. How many sexually active people are there in the United Kingdom? Do all sexually active people practise safe sex by using a barrier method of contraception such as condoms in the United Kingdom? A survey could be used to give an indication of how many. A questionnaire could then be devised to distribute to sexually active adults in order to find out what brands of sexual protection (condom, femidom or dental dam) are used. This kind of survey would try to find out when people used protection, when they were least likely and most likely to use protection, and how much money was spent on sexual protection per week. The information might be useful in a health promotion context:

- If running a safe sex campaign in a family planning clinic.
- Or in a genito-urinary clinic.
- When identifying specific health promotion needs used in identifying trends in patient/client behaviour.
- When considering social policy issues relating to such health issues as national trends in the development of HIV/AIDS.

First, the population that is to be sampled must be targeted, for example, consenting adults over the age of eighteen years. Note that this would not give you any information about those under eighteen, as they are not part of the target population.

Box 4.2

The questionnaire

This survey is attempting to find out about the use of barrier methods of contraception/protection. Your answers will be treated in confidence and will help us plan health care services. Please indicate your responses by placing a cross in the box next to the answer you think *best represents your answer:* (1) strongly agree, (2) agree, (3) not sure, (4) disagree, (5) strongly disagree.

1   I use the following types of barrier protection?

	Always				Never
	1	2	3	4	5
None	☐	☐	☐	☐	☐
Condom	☐	☐	☐	☐	☐
Femidom	☐	☐	☐	☐	☐
Dental dam	☐	☐	☐	☐	☐
Cap (Dutch cap)	☐	☐	☐	☐	☐

2   When are you most likely to use sexual protection?

	Agree				Disagree
	1	2	3	4	5
I never use barrier methods of sexual protection	☐	☐	☐	☐	☐
I sometimes use protection when I remember	☐	☐	☐	☐	☐
I use a condom every time I have anal penetrative sex	☐	☐	☐	☐	☐
To avoid pregnancy	☐	☐	☐	☐	☐
Allergic to latex	☐	☐	☐	☐	☐
To avoid getting a sexually transmitted disease	☐	☐	☐	☐	☐

3   Please indicate your circumstances: which of the following categories applies to you? Tick those that do.

Single
Married or cohabiting
Living with spouse
Living with partner
I have many sexual partners
I have one sexual partner

Thank you for completing this questionnaire. Please return it in the enclosed pre-paid envelope. Your responses will be treated in confidence.

Questionnaires: the reality

A common misconception about questionnaires is that they are often considered an easy tool to use in research. In reality, the use of questionnaires requires a great deal of time and effort in terms of careful planning, ordering and sequencing of the questions and the responses in order to obtain relevant data. As with most research, we need to address questions of design early in the study. When using questionnaires not only do we have issues of the sample to consider (see Chapter 3) but also specific issues that concern the questionnaire, for example:

- When should the questionnaire be administered and how: by mail, in person, by telephone interview or face to face, e-mail or Internet?
- Where should the questionnaire be administered and by whom?
- How will the questions be arranged in terms of sequencing, degree of ease or difficulty?
- Are the questions to be addressed in the questionnaire intrusive, do they pry into sensitive or private areas of people's lives, such as death and dying or sexual persuasion or activities, and are they likely to cause offence or distress to respondents?

The importance of the points raised above is that they all have the potential to bias the answers that you receive. If for example you are asking questions about sexual behaviour, whether you use telephone or face-to-face questioning is likely to alter the results, as is the gender of the respondent in relation to the interviewer. Any bias will introduce error, which will make interpreting the results harder.

In addition to the considerations above you will need to think about how the information will be handled and stored, remembering that many countries have laws to protect respondent or subject confidentiality and the use to which data can be put. This is also important for all types of study where personal data are collected. Many countries have specific legislation that covers how data can be stored and how they can be used. You must make sure that your systems of data handling conform to the law of whichever country you are working in.

When we want to use a questionnaire to produce quantitative data it is important that all our variables and the responses are given in a form that can be analysed using statistics. This means that the answers should come in the form of numbers. If you intend to use a computer to help with the analysis it is also important for the variables to be given codes that the computer finds easy to handle. When preparing data for analysis each case should be given a row on a table and each variable a column (see Table 5.1). Most data from questionnaires tend to be either ordinal or nominal scale data.

Asking questions

When designing a questionnaire there are also issues concerning the formulation of the questions. You need to consider how the questions will impact upon the answers.

Box 4.3

Leading questions

Try asking your friends or colleagues about how they rate the quality of their lunch. Can you lead them to suggest in general their lunch is (1) poor or (2) good? Which types of question are the best at leading?
Look at the sample questionnaire. Which of the questions do you think are leading? How would you rephrase them?

Leading questions

A leading question is a question that leads the respondent to a particular answer. By using leading questions experimenters have been able to demonstrate effects on guessing measurements, past personal experience and recently witnessed events. In everyday language we often use leading questions, and as such, when designing questionnaires, leading questions are often easy to include by mistake. Things to watch out for in particular are an implied direction when asking a respondent to put a value on something. If we were to ask people to indicate their degree of agreement with the statement 'Condoms are a good form of contraception' more people would tend to agree with the statement. If, however, we asked the same people to indicate their agreement with the statement 'Condoms are a poor form of contraception' we would also find more people tending to agree with the statement. In both cases we have led the respondents to the answer. Emotive words should also be avoided. Studies have shown, for example, that when people were asked to estimate the speed at which two cars collided, the actual speed suggested depends on the word used (smashed, crashed, etc.) to describe the collision.

Ordering

Care needs to be taken when ordering questions; in general, the basic principle is that the ordering should be logical and that the questionnaire should appear structured and clear. For example, if you were asking people about their experience as a diabetic it would not be logical to ask questions about how they delivered insulin before asking if the respondents were insulin-dependent. Structure can be achieved through grouping similar questions together, either by subject or by type of answer.

Sensitive questions should be placed towards the end of the questionnaire, as they can cause people to refuse to answer. An early refusal tends to lead the respondent to abandon the questionnaire.

Questions about the respondents' personal details should also come at the end. Asking for this information at the start tends to make respondents concerned about your commitment to their confidentiality.

Scales

When asking respondents a question we quite often give them a range of options so that they can indicate where their answer lies according to a scale. In the example questionnaire above (Box 4.2) we used a scale for respondents to express their frequency of use of differing types of contraceptive and also a scale for respondents to indicate their level of agreement with certain statements. There are a range of scales of this type; we will now discuss three of them.

The scale most commonly used is the Likert scale, named after Rensis Likert, who invented it. The Likert scale measures the extent to which a person agrees or disagrees with the question. The most common scale is 1 to 5. Often the scale will be (1) strongly disagree, (2) disagree, (3) not sure, (4) agree and (5) strongly agree.

One common problem with using a scale which is based on an odd (five) number of options is that it always provides the option of choosing the middle point. Often it is easier for respondents to take this 'easy' option than to struggle to make a decision. Using a scale with an even number of options (four or six, for example) forces respondents to choose between tending to agree or tending to disagree. There are two problems here. Some individuals may be genuinely neutral, and using an even number of options forces on them a choice they may not agree with; and psychologically individuals may assume that the scale has a 0. Thus if you present a scale of 1–4, people will select 2 as a neutral value, as on a normal number line 2 is half-way between 0 and 4. In general it is probably better to opt for an odd number of options and accept that those people who select the neutral option probably do not have a strong opinion.

Another type of scale is the Thurstone scale. A Thurstone scale uses just two points: agree and disagree. When using Thurstone scales, it is usual to ask several related questions that can be used to produce an overall score for an individual respondent. The overall score can then be compared with that for the sample as a whole, or used so that differing populations are compared. A common example of the use of Thurstone scales is in psychometric tests. Psychometric tests test aptitude and attitude. You might expect to complete such a test as part of a job interview.

An alternative approach is to use semantic differential scales, which are good for investigating phenomena such as attitude and values. A semantic differential scale is based on opposite points of view, or potential emotions about a subject or concept. The respondent is asked to indicate where on the scale he or she sits. We may, for example, be investigating people's work environment. We ask questions concerning how they felt about aspects of the environment, and the response scale may range from helpful, nurturing, happy to unsupportive, blocking, toxic, dysfunctional.

In Table 4.1 the concept is 'day surgery'; patients are asked to indicate where on the scale they lie. You would probably want to ask more questions to get a good overview of an individual's impressions of day surgery. Note that there is no consistent negative end of the scale. This helps to persuade the respondents to think about their answers.

Table 4.1   A patient's responses when asked to consider day surgery (questions asked pre-operatively)

Exciting	1	2	3	4	5	6	Boring
Frightening	1	2	3	4	5	6	Calming
Useful	1	2	3	4	5	6	Useless
Fast	1	2	3	4	5	6	Slow

Box 4.4

Writing questions

- Develop five questions using a Likert scale to measure the quality of primary health care service used by your peers.
- Ask at least three of your peers to respond to the questions you have devised and ask each to indicate to you how clear they think the questions are.
- Do you need to revise the questions?
- Did the questions you asked appear to measure what you intended?

Validity and reliability of questionnaires in statistical analysis

Questionnaires should be seen as measurement tools, just as we view a thermometer or a ruler. As with these tools, we need to ask how valid the measures are, that is, do they really measure what we think they do, and reliability, that is, will the same result be returned over time and if administering the questionnaire were to repeated?

With questionnaires, rather than dealing with the validity and reliability of instruments, the issues centre on the interaction of the tool with individuals, whose responses can change depending on their circumstances. Unlike the measurement of physical responses, the types of circumstances and level of impact are not easy to measure, and much effort needs to be devoted to ensuring that a questionnaire is reliable and valid. As this book concerns quantitative analysis, below we explore the concepts of reliability and validity as they relate to the quantitative analysis of data from questionnaires.

Reliability

Reliability involves two main concepts: consistency over time (or stability), for example, if you record results from one group of individuals do you get the same results if you measure the same group a few days or weeks later, and will these results demonstrate internal consistency? This means, will this questionnaire produce similar responses under repeated conditions?

To test for stability (consistency over time) it is possible to perform a retest reliability test to show the extent to which the same scores are obtained when the instrument (questionnaire) is used with the same subjects twice. This test produces a **reliability coefficient** that indicates how small the differences are between the scores. The coefficient ranges between 0.00 and 1.00, the higher the score the better. The Pearson correlation coefficient is often used. (This coefficient is discussed in Chapter 16.)

The internal consistency factor of the concept of reliability relates directly to the way in which the questions in the questionnaire designed to measure an attribute consistently and nothing else. This means that all the items on the scale are accurate in their focus on data collection and can be seen to be all working in the same direction. Similar respondents will tend to give the same pattern of answers if the questionnaire is internally consistent. If we introduced a question that had little to do with the other questions, the internal consistency would decrease. For example, if in the survey on sexual health we introduced a question such as 'To what extent do you agree with the statement "Ice cream is nice"?' we would not expect the answers to be at all related to respondents' previous answers and therefore internal consistency would be lost.

There are various methods of determining internal consistency. The most common is the **Cronbach alpha reliability coefficient** test. Again the coefficient ranges between 0.00 and 1.00, the higher the score the better. In general, a score above 0.80 indicates a high level of internal consistency. The score's value is, however, related to the number of questions asked. As you ask more questions the score will tend to increase.

Validity

Validity refers to the extent to which a questionnaire measures what it is supposed to measure by obtaining data relevant to the topic which is being measured, for example, if the topic area for measurement is degrees of sexual libido, how can degrees of libido be measured whilst ensuring that measuring deviance or sexual perversion does not become the focus of the study? There are several different forms and measures of validity. We discuss some of these below.

Content validity

This is a weak form of validity and concerns the **representativeness** of the questions, in other words do the questions adequately sample the content being investigated? One way to ensure that questions asked of respondents are valid, pertinent and measurable is to conduct a thorough literature review of the topic before constructing the questionnaire.

Face validity

This is obtained through asking a member of the lay public to assess questions for accuracy and completeness. If you want to assess whether the content reflects the subject matter, you can use a panel of experts or a group of peers. This is often termed a *focus group*, as the panel or group shares the same focus of interest in the topic being investigated.

Criterion-related validity

This is a strong form of validity, as criterion-related validity measures the ability to compare equality to another already validated measuring instrument or questionnaire. This instrument has shown itself to be accurate in obtaining or measuring data.

Predictive validity

This refers to the ability of the questionnaire to predict some criterion observed at a future date with the data collected on the criterion variable at a different time but on the same subjects. For example A-level results and end-of-year examinations.

Construct validity

This is the most difficult type of validity to achieve. The question is: what construct is the instrument actually measuring? The more abstract the construct the harder this is, because of the absence of objective criteria to measure the construct. For example grief, role conflict, empathy, etc.

Known-groups technique

This means you can use two groups who have a shared experience in whom you would expect to see a difference, for example, measuring fear of childbirth in pregnancy. You could, for example, choose a group of primaparas and a group of multiparas. Your guess or research hunch is that the first-time-pregnant group is more likely to express fear of the labour process than those who have had several births. This may be reflected in the scores.

How can questionnaires be analysed?

Having obtained your data, you will want to analyse it. Most phenomena measured by questionnaires use either the **nominal** (categories) or **ordinal** scales (see Chapter 3) and these will affect the type of descriptive and analytical statistics that you can use. Chapter 6 discusses how data measured on the ordinal scale can be described and Chapter 7 how they can be displayed. Chapters 14 and 15 describe statistical tests that are particularly useful for the type of data gathered by questionnaires.

Having read this chapter and completed the exercises, you should be familiar with the following ideas and concepts:

- When to use a questionnaire
- Types of question not to ask
- Basic aspects of questionnaire design
- The concept of reliability
- The concept of validity
- Response scales

Exercises

1 For the study on the walk-in clinic presented in Chapter 5, review the questions and decide which, if any, are leading. How would you improve on this questionnaire?

2 Identify three studies from the literature that use questionnaires. For each study: (a) decide what the research question was and why a questionnaire was appropriate, (b) review how the validity and reliability of the questionnaire were considered.

3 Using a topic that interests you, draw up a short (six questions) questionnaire using questions that are not leading. Ask a colleague or friend to assess the quality of your questions. Do they lead? Are they clear and unambiguous?

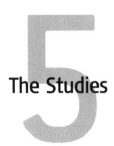

The Studies

In this chapter we provide the background and data from two hypothetical studies, one from a clinical trial and the other from a questionnaire. In some of the exercises at the end of each chapter we ask you to analyse data from these studies. If you work your way through all the exercises you will have completed a basic analysis of these data sets and be able to draw some conclusions and be in a better position to analyse critically this and other studies. These studies have been devised to be relevant to modern health care as well as to stimulate your interest and enjoyment of data analysis. Please note the main purpose of this questionnaire is to provide data for you to analyse, therefore we have not presented data from all sections of the presented studies.

The questionnaire study

This questionnaire concerns the sexual health of individuals who presented for advice at a walk-in clinic in central London. It was partly introduced in Chapter 4. Here we show the extended version, although for the sake of simplicity we have reduced the extent of some of the questions.

The aim of this study is to provide basic information as to the sexual behaviour of individuals of differing sex, age and ethnic group who used the walk-in clinic. The study was initiated because the clinical leader considered that a large proportion of the clients were presenting with symptoms that related to sexual heath and she was considering putting in a bid for funds to support the employment of a specialist in this area. The study is largely descriptive and exploratory in nature.

   The population of the study is all those individuals who could potentially use the walk-in centre. The sample is made up of those that actually did enter the clinic and complete the questionnaire.

The questionnaire

This survey is attempting to find out about the use of the walk-in clinic in relation to sexual health. Your answers will be treated in confidence and will help us plan health care services. Please indicate your responses by placing a cross in the box next to the answer you think best represents your answer.

1   What made you attend the walk-in centre today?

	Agree				Disagree
	1	2	3	4	5
Location	☐	☐	☐	☐	☐
Availability	☐	☐	☐	☐	☐
Access to medical staff	☐	☐	☐	☐	☐
Access to nursing staff	☐	☐	☐	☐	☐
Emergency treatment required	☐	☐	☐	☐	☐

2   What symptoms are you experiencing? Please tick the *one* you feel best describes your symptoms

Headache
Chills/shakes
Temperature
Lack of appetite
Feeling generally unwell all over
Cough
Pain/soreness in chest
Faintness
Collapse
Pain or difficulty passing urine
Discharge from penis
Discharge from vagina

3   Which of the following descriptions best represents your sex life? (Please tick.)

   (a)   Very active (I have sex more than five times per week)
   (b)   Active (I have sex between once and five times per week)
   (c)   Not very active (I have sex less than once per week)
   (d)   Non-existent

4 Please indicate how many sexual partners you have shared sex with
   in the past month.

5 My most frequent choice of barrier protection is: (Please tick one)

None
Condom
Femidom
Dental dam
Cap (Dutch cap)

6 When are you most likely to use sexual protection?

	Agree 1	2	3	4	Disagree 5
I never use barrier methods of sexual protection	☐	☐	☐	☐	☐
I sometimes use protection when I remember	☐	☐	☐	☐	☐
I use protection (put a condom on) if I do not know my sexual partner very well	☐	☐	☐	☐	☐
I use protection (put a condom on) when I think I am going to climax	☐	☐	☐	☐	☐
I use a condom every time I have oral sex	☐	☐	☐	☐	☐
I use a condom every time I have vaginal penetrative sex	☐	☐	☐	☐	☐
I use a condom every time I have anal penetrative sex	☐	☐	☐	☐	☐
To avoid pregnancy	☐	☐	☐	☐	☐
To avoid getting a sexually transmitted disease	☐	☐	☐	☐	☐

7 What puts you off using sexual protection?

	Agree 1	2	3	4	Disagree 5
Not very comfortable	☐	☐	☐	☐	☐
Loss of sensation/cannot feel anything	☐	☐	☐	☐	☐
Too fiddly to have to open packets	☐	☐	☐	☐	☐
Cost	☐	☐	☐	☐	☐

By the time the packet is open
　the moment has gone　　　　　　☐　☐　☐　☐　☐
Need to use a lubricant as well　☐　☐　☐　☐　☐
Have to plan sex in advance　　　☐　☐　☐　☐　☐
Allergic to latex　　　　　　　　☐　☐　☐　☐　☐

8　How much money do you spend, on average, on sexual protection per week? Please indicate which category applies to you, using a tick:

£0
£0–£5
£5–£10
£10–15
I get them free

9　My age group is: Please indicate which category applies to you using a tick.

16–24	25–34	35–44	45–54	55–64	65–74	75–100
☐	☐	☐	☐	☐	☐	☐

11　I consider my sexual orientation to be:

Heterosexual male
Heterosexual female
Gay (homosexual) male
Gay (lesbian) female
Bisexual male
Bisexual female
Asexual

12　I consider my ethnic background to be:

(a)　African
(b)　Asian
(c)　European

(The questionnaire has been simplified for the purposes of this book.)

When entering data into charts and computers it is often easier to use a line for each subject and enter values across the rows for the variables measured. Often codes will be used to simplify the data entry. In Table 5.1 we have used the following codes. For gender we have used M for male and F for female. For sexual activity we have used a code from 1 (very active) to 4 (non-existent). For 'barrier choice' we have used codes 1–5 for

Table 5.1   The data from the questionnaire

					Questions			
		13	12 Ethic group	3 Sexual activity	4	5 Barrier choice	7 Reason not	2	9
Individual	Sex				Partners			Presentation	Age
1	F	E	3	1	1	1	1	22
2	F	E	2	2	2	5	7	28
3	F	E	1	8	2	7	4	21
4	F	AS	2	1	2	1	9	26
5	F	AS	4	0	0	5	12	27
6	F	AS	2	1	0	7	6	30
7	F	AS	4	0	2	5	5	29
8	F	AS	2	2	0	5	12	23
9	F	E	4	0	1	3	10	21
10	F	E	2	1	0	2	9	32
11	F	E	1	1	1	2	3	18
12	F	E	1	1	3	7	10	24
13	F	A	1	3	5	6	12	23
14	F	A	2	4	1	1	7	23
15	F	A	1	1	5	3	12	20
16	F	A	3	0	2	5	1	36
17	F	E	1	4	0	5	2	20
18	F	E	3	1	0	1	5	23
19	F	E	4	0	2	3	3	24
20	F	E	4	2	3	3	3	20
21	F	E	3	0	2	1	12	34
22	F	E	3	1	1	7	12	25
23	M	E	1	12	2	4	2	19
24	M	E	2	1	1	6	1	53
25	M	E	3	2	2	3	1	26
26	M	A	2	1	2	4	5	29
27	M	A	3	2	1	4	7	58
28	M	A	3	2	1	2	7	37
29	M	A	1	12	0	5	8	22
30	M	A	2	3	1	4	11	23
31	M	A	4	1	0	4	3	36
32	M	A	2	1	1	5	8	25
33	M	AS	2	1	2	6	12	44
34	M	AS	4	1	2	6	11	41
35	M	E	2	1	2	6	2	22
36	M	E	4	1	1	4	8	27
37	M	E	1	18	2	8	11	35
38	M	E	2	2	1	1	11	35
39	M	E	2	2	1	8	7	22
40	M	E	1	1	1	2	8	39

for the most used protection the participant selected. 1 is the first response possible (none) and 5 the last (Cap). For question 7 we have used a similar system to that used for barrier choice where 1 is the first option and 8 the last. For the presentation type we have also used the same system as for questions 5 and 7, with 1 equivalent to 'headache' and 12 to 'discharge from vagina'.

The clinical trial

This experimental trial looks at the ability of the novel drug Symphadiol* to help increase weight loss in individuals who are trying to lose weight using a calorie-controlled diet. This clinical trial is being organised by Spinto**, a drug company, which is active in this field. Spinto have recruited individuals to take part in their study using a network of dieters' groups. Individuals were invited to take part by Spinto's clinical trials specialist nurse, who will conduct the study, with the support of local GPs and Spinto's dietician.

The aim of the experiment is to test the hypothesis that a daily dose of Symphadiol enhances weight loss, in clinically obese individuals, compared with just using a calorie-controlled diet. It was decided to select men between the ages of twenty two and forty for the study. It was also decided to look at the impact of exercise in conjunction with Symphadiol.

The population in this study are all healthy (other than their obesity) obese male individuals who are sufficiently motivated to lose weight to join a diet network. The individuals must not be taking any medication, except that required for minor ailments.

In total 120 males were recruited between the ages of twenty two to forty. Each participant was given a health check prior to the start of the study. Their heights were recorded and they received educational material and diets giving details of a calorie-restricted diet (1,500 kcal), which they declared they would follow. All the men attended weekly diet networks where they received support and encouragement from their fellow dieters and the clinical trials specialist nurse. Those individuals following an exercise regime also attended a gym and completed the equivalent of thirty minutes' cycling (18 km) three times per week.

The participants were distributed randomly to four experimental groups:

1　Calorie-controlled diet and placebo.
2　Calorie-controlled diet and 35mg Symphadiol orally OD.
3　Exercise regime, calorie-controlled diet and placebo.
4　Exercise regime, calorie-controlled diet and 35 mg Symphadiol orally OD.

---

* Symphadiol is a fictitious name
** Spinto is a fictitious name

Table 5.2 shows the results for sixty of the participants, fifteen from each group.

Table 5.2 The data from the clinical trial

Individual	Age	Height (cm)	Group	Weight loss (kg)
1	32	159	1	23
2	35	174	1	16
3	35	188	1	28
4	33	174	1	12
5	30	195	1	8
6	38	195	1	17
7	39	176	1	−1
8	36	193	1	16
9	31	159	1	20
10	38	170	1	1
11	33	177	1	6
12	38	167	1	7
13	34	184	1	−3
14	37	193	1	10
15	39	181	1	14
16	31	186	2	23
17	32	182	2	18
18	36	158	2	8
19	38	170	2	12
20	31	184	2	15
21	36	176	2	0
22	35	158	2	1
23	30	169	2	9
24	34	175	2	16
25	37	188	2	15
26	37	188	2	10
27	34	195	2	6
28	37	182	2	4
29	34	171	2	0
30	38	198	2	18
31	32	181	3	20
32	34	169	3	13
33	34	181	3	22
34	34	190	3	24
35	37	193	3	23
36	30	177	3	11
37	35	158	3	10
38	35	181	3	18
39	37	181	3	18
40	37	183	3	25
41	25	176	3	7
42	35	172	3	11
43	38	192	3	18
44	35	194	3	20
45	30	179	3	14
46	35	171	4	25

(Continued)

Table 5.2 (Continued)

Individual	Age	Height (cm)	Group	Weight loss (kg)
47	38	179	4	27
48	36	178	4	28
49	31	188	4	17
50	33	180	4	21
51	35	184	4	13
52	37	173	4	5
53	39	176	4	5
54	38	170	4	6
55	32	190	4	26
56	32	152	4	6
57	37	182	4	10
58	35	175	4	10
59	34	180	4	8
60	32	162	4	22

Please remember that these studies are hypothetical and are designed to help you practise. As with all skills, if you don't practise they won't develop. Use these data how you wish, discuss your results with colleagues and have fun.

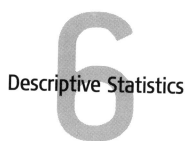

Descriptive Statistics

Areas of learning covered in this chapter

How are   data described and summarised?
What are   measures of central tendency and dispersion?
How are   measures of central tendency and dispersion calculated?
Which   measure of central tendency do I use and when?

We use descriptive statistics when we want to describe what our data look like, or what their most common features might be. Descriptive statistics are used to summarise our data. After all, if you were to present all the data that had been gathered in a study your audience would probably soon lose interest.

Descriptive statistics can thus be used to give the reader a summary of the data you have collected. Producing descriptive statistics will also help us to understand whether we have captured the sort of data we want. For example, using the variable 'age', descriptive statistics could demonstrate whether we had captured the range of ages we wanted. Did we accidentally include too many young people? Or perhaps a few people in the sample were much older than the rest of the cases. Descriptive statistics allow us to get a feel for the data, to appreciate their common features and any unusual features. This is nothing new, we do it to understand behaviour and actions all the time. For example, a common question in lifestyle surveys is 'How much time you give to exercise in a day?' Obviously you are not expected to write that on Tuesday you spent forty minutes, Thursday thirty seven minutes, etc. You will be expected (or even asked) to give an average. Say, for example, on average, you exercise forty five minutes a day. But some days, when you are tired, you may exercise for just twenty minutes. Alternatively on a particularly energetic day you may do eighty minutes. Then you would have exercised anywhere between twenty and eighty minutes. In this example the researcher is asking you to summarise your day-to-day exercise level and provide a descriptive statistic, the average. Descriptive statistics allow us to summarise detailed data in a manner that can be interpreted quickly and easily.

Box 6.1

Descriptive statistics

Think about the statistics that you have heard or seen in the last week. Why do you think they were quoted?

Descriptive statistics are used in many aspects of health care. They are, in fact, the most common type of statistic you are likely to encounter. Descriptive statistics are used to manage, to monitor and to evaluate health services and the people who work in them. This is why understanding descriptive statistics is so important for those who work in a health care setting. Descriptive statistics are usually divided into two types: (1) measures of central tendency (typical value), the mean, the mode and the median, (2) measures of variability about the typical value (measures of dispersion) – range, inter-quartile range, standard deviation and variance.

Measures of central tendency

Mean

Arithmetic mean – we usually call this the average. To calculate the average time we spend in a gym in a month we would take the times spent during each visit, add them together and divide by the number of visits. Table 6.1, for example, displays the time that an individual (Mr Armstrong) spent in the gym during the month of July.

Table 6.1 Time spent by an individual at the gym during July

Visit	Time spent (minutes)
1	62
2	34
3	50
4	40
5	58
6	48
7	38
8	60
9	58
10	45
11	53
12	32

To calculate the mean:

$$\text{Mean} = \frac{32 + 34 + 38 + 40 + 45 + 48 + 50 + 53 + 58 + 58 + 60 + 62}{12} = \frac{578}{12} = 48.16$$

Minutes spent in each visit

Total number of visits

So the average (mean) length of time spent in the gym is 48.16 minutes. You can see that this score of 48.16 minutes falls approximately in the centre of our data, with six visit times less than this and six greater. This is not always the case with the mean, however.

Box 6.2

Calculators

Most statistics involve only the use of calculations that can be carried out on a basic calculator. Most calculators also have a facility that will allow you to perform the basic statistical calculations faster, and once data sets become large use a computer package. Look on your calculator for some of the symbols described above. If your calculator has a statistical function, they normally can be found below the function buttons.

Unfortunately for those just starting out in the world of statistics, being a branch of mathematics, statistical tests are often represented as a formula. Understanding them is like learning another language. It is the use of symbols which usually leaves people convinced they cannot understand statistics. So to introduce a few:

x An individual case, like one visit to the gym.

n The number of cases (x) so twelve visits to the gym means that $n = 12$.

$\sum$ 'The sum of', e.g. all the xs added up. In the case above, $\sum x. = 578$.

$\bar{x}$ The symbol for the mean.

Another way of describing how to calculate the mean other than using words is:

$$\bar{x} = \frac{\sum x}{n}$$

(Note: this is the formula used when calculating the mean for a sample from a population.)

If you have problems following a statistical formula, write out each symbol in words. Thus for the mean we have:

$$Mean = \frac{The\ sum\ of\ the\ cases}{The\ number\ of\ cases}$$

There is one disadvantage with the mean. It can be misleading when some of the values are unusually small or large. If, for example, Mr Armstrong on one day stayed in the gym for just five minutes, adding this value to our data would affect the average score, making the average 44.85 minutes.

Box 6.3

In the example from the gym, the sample is one month's visits; the population would be all of Mr Armstrong's visits. When dealing with whole populations statisticians use different symbols to distinguish between samples and populations. In addition, when calculating statistics, the equations slightly change. This book will focus on statistics that concern samples from populations, but do be aware that there are subtle differences. Some symbols used when talking about populations:

N The population size.

μ The population mean.

σ The standard deviation (see below) of the population.

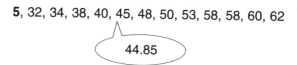

5, 32, 34, 38, 40, 45, 48, 50, 53, 58, 58, 60, 62

44.85

You can see how this unusual score of 5 has made the mean much lower, therefore it is not a true reflection of the central point. These extreme values are called *outliers*.

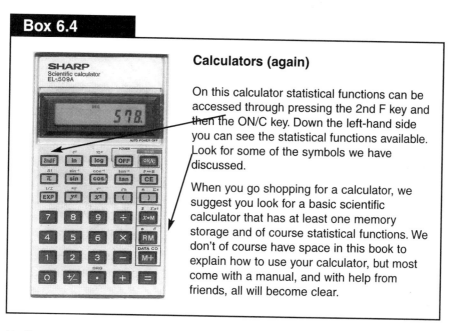

Box 6.4

SHARP
Scientific calculator
EL-509A

Calculators (again)

On this calculator statistical functions can be accessed through pressing the 2nd F key and then the ON/C key. Down the left-hand side you can see the statistical functions available. Look for some of the symbols we have discussed.

When you go shopping for a calculator, we suggest you look for a basic scientific calculator that has at least one memory storage and of course statistical functions. We don't of course have space in this book to explain how to use your calculator, but most come with a manual, and with help from friends, all will become clear.

Median

The median helps to solve the problem of outliers because, rather than use all the values to calculate the statistic of central tendency, it uses only the value that sits in the middle of the data. It is the physical centre. So far, we have put our data in ascending order. This is essential to do when calculating the median.

If we take our two examples of exercise time and include the low value, we can see that it has very little impact on the median even when it only occurs at one end.

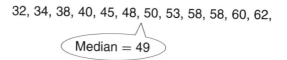

32, 34, 38, 40, 45, 48, 50, 53, 58, 58, 60, 62,

Median = 49

5, 32, 34, 38, 40, 45, 48, 50, 53, 58, 58, 60, 62,

Median = 48

The extreme value only moves the median by 1. Where the middle falls between two values, it is necessary to add the two middle numbers and divide by 2, for example:

$$\frac{48 + 50}{2} = 49$$

Box 6.5

Collect a sample of the pulse rate from fifteen individuals.

- Calculate the mean.
- Calculate the median.

So why don't we hear or see the median being quoted more often? The simple answer is that it is not widely understood by the general public. But also, because the median is not arithmetically based, it cannot easily be manipulated or used in further calculations.

Mode

The mode is the most frequently occurring value, so from our data set we can see it is 58.

32, 34, 38, 40, 45, 48, 50, 53, **58, 58**, 60, 62,

The mode shows the most common value. One of the advantages of the mode is that it can be used on both continuous and nominal data, whereas the mean and median can be used only on continuous data.

At times, therefore, it is the only option as a measure of central tendency. For example, one question a lifestyle survey asked was where students would primarily go for family planning advice:

- GP   5
- Practice nurse   4
- Family planning clinic   6
- Friends   8
- Chemist   2
- Nowhere   2

So the most commonly occurring category was friends, with eight scores. For the data in this list, the mean and median would have no meaning.

Choosing a measure of central tendency

It is most common to use the mean, as it is the most sensitive. The mean considers all the values of each case in the distribution, as described above. The mean is arithmetically based, so it can be used in further calculations. However, it can only be used on data of interval or ratio level of measurement and is easily distorted by outliers.

Box 6.6

Choosing measures

Ask a sample of your friends how often (each week) they eat chocolate. For this sample, find:

- The mean.
- The mode.
- The median.

Which do you think best represents the typical value? Why?

The median, which does not take account of the values of the cases, is unaffected by outliers and is suitable for ordinal/ranked data. Where the mean is distorted by the presence of outliers the median should be used.

The mode can be used on data of all levels of measurement but is most useful for categorical data. On a normal distribution the mode, median and mean should all be the same. It is also possible to have more than one mode.

Box 6.7

Choosing a measure of central tendency

Measure	When to use	When not to use
Mean	Interval or ratio data	Categorical data Ordinal data
	For most data sets, where the cases are more or less symmetrically distributed about the mean	When there are outliers or the data are heavily skewed
	Where the measure is going to be used in further calculations	
Median	Interval, ratio or ordinal data, Data heavily skewed, mean distorted by outliers.	When the measure will be used in further calculations
Mode	Categorical	Ordinal data

In many circumstances there is no right or wrong measure of central tendency and people tend to opt for the arithmetic mean because they are familiar with it. Remember, the main point of descriptive statistics is to communicate information. You should choose the measure that conveys the information in the best possible way and does not mislead the audience.

Measures of dispersion

So far, we have looked at central values. Now we are going to explore statistics which tell us how different our scores within a sample are. Dispersion is the term given to those measures that tell us about the level of variability with the data. If there were no variation in populations there would be little need for statistics.

We asked two groups of students, one group full-time and one part-time, how old they were when they had their first sexual experience with another person.

Group A   14, 15, 18, 22, 23 = $\bar{x}_A$ 18.4

Group B   17, 18, 19, 19, 20 = $\bar{x}_B$ 18.6

This subscript tells us that the mean is that of group A

Whilst the means are the same it is obvious that there is a difference in the variability of the values of the cases with the groups.

In terms of using the statistics to develop health care practices, knowing the variability of values is as important as knowing the mean. After all, if shoe manufacturers only made shoes for people with average-size feet they would soon go out of business. We want to know about the variability in patients' health that we will encounter and in their behaviours.

Range

One measure of dispersion is the range. To calculate this you subtract the lowest score from the highest, so the range of group A is:

$$23 - 14 = 9$$

The range of group B is:

$$20 - 17 = 3$$

This tells us that for group A scores are spread over nine units, but for group B they cover only three. This means that group A has a greater range of values in its cases. The range is a quick and easy way of estimating the level of variation within your sample, but beware of outliers.

Inter-quartile range

To deal with outliers an alternative is to use the inter-quartile range (IQR). A quartile, as the name suggests, is derived by quartering the data set. The data are placed in ascending order and divided into four quarters. The numbers at the boundaries of these quarters are known as quartiles. The IQR is really the range for the middle fifty per cent of the data. It is calculated by locating the upper value of the first quartile (first 25 per cent of the cases) and subtracting it from the upper value of the third quartile. In the following example, we asked a group of teenagers for how many years they thought it was safe to take the contraceptive pill (Q, quartile).

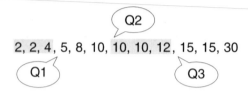

The range is 28 but it is affected by the case with the value of 30. There are 12 cases in the set of data, so there will be three cases in each quartile. At the end of the first quartile (first 25 per cent of the cases) the value is 4. At the end of the third quartile (first 75 per cent of the cases) the value is 12. The difference between these values (8) is the IQR.

Box 6.8

Calculate the IQR for the data you gathered for the exercise in Box 6.6.

Whilst the range and IQR say something about spread, they ignore any concept of the level of deviation from the central tendency. The standard deviation (SD), however, uses each score to calculate spread and how far each score is, in standard terms, away from the mean.

The standard deviation and variance

The two most common measures of dispersion that indicate the amount of deviation from the mean are the standard deviation and the variance. Most quoted in describing data is the standard deviation, whilst the variance is used in many statistical tests.

The standard deviation is a measure of the variation in the data that evaluates how much each case deviates from the mean. If the mean is say 6 and an individual case is 8 then the deviation is 2. Whilst this is easy enough and takes care of the deviation part of the statistic it's really the standard bit that is important. To obtain a standard deviation we take all the deviations and look at them in relation to the size of the mean. This is important because a deviation of 2 is of much less importance if the mean is 110 than if it is 8.

Table 6.2   Age at first sexual experience (with another person).

Case	1	2	3	4	5	6	7	8	9	10
Age of first sexual experience	14	15	17	18	18	19	19	20	22	23

The formula for the standard deviation is given below. It looks complex but it really involves quite straightforward maths. We will take you through the formula step by step, using the data in Table 6.2.

$$s = \sqrt{\frac{\sum (x - \bar{x})^2}{n - 1}}$$

s is the symbol for the standard deviation and s^2 is the symbol for the variance. The variance is simply the standard deviation squared. The calculation steps are outlined below:

Step 1:   Calculate the mean.
Step 2:   Subtract the mean from each value $x - \bar{x}$

$14 - 18.5 = \quad -4.5$
$15 - 18.5 = \quad -3.5$
$17 - 18.5 = \quad -1.5$
$18 - 18.5 = \quad -0.5$
$18 - 18.5 = \quad -0.5$
$19 - 18.5 = \quad 0.5$
$19 - 18.5 = \quad 0.5$
$20 - 18.5 = \quad 1.5$
$22 - 18.5 = \quad 3.5$
$23 - 18.5 = \quad 4.5$

Step 3:   Square each answer obtained in step 2.
Step 4:   Add up all the answers to step 3. This value is called the sum of squares.
Step 5:   Minus 1 from the size of your sample ($n - 1$).
Step 6:   Divide the value found in step 4 by the value calculated in step 5:

Box 6.9

Standard deviation

We asked a group of thirty people to keep a record of how many times they thought about sex in a day. The results were: 7, 7, 8, 10, 10, 12, 14, 15, 16, 17, 18, 20, 20, 21, 21, 21, 22, 23, 24, 26, 28, 28, 30, 32, 34, 35, 36, 38, 40, 42. Is the mean a good measure of central tendency and how spread out are the results from it?

$$\frac{\sum(x-\bar{x})^2}{n-1} = \frac{70.5}{9} = 7.83$$

This is called the **variance**.

Step 7:　Find the square root of the value obtained in step 6 to determine the value of one standard deviation:

$$\sqrt{7.83} = 2.80$$

Thus the standard deviation of our sample was 2.80.

If you want to do a statistical test, be cautious of data sets, where the square of the standard deviation (the variance) is much larger than the mean (two times), where the variance is small in relation to the mean, or where the variance equals the mean. These are indications that the data set might have a more complex form and need to be handled in a particular way.

It is important when you quote a mean always to give a measure of the dispersion. A measure of the mean without a measure of dispersion is difficult to interpret; the sample size should also be included. Remember these important facts when you next hear the average house price or salary quoted in the press or on television.

Which measure of dispersion should you quote? In general, when you use a mean give a standard deviation, if you quote the median give the interquartile range. Don't be modest with your use of measures of dispersion; remember, descriptive statistics are about describing your results to your audience.

Box 6.10

Central tendency and measure of dispersion

Type of data	Measure of central tendency	Measure of dispersion
For most data sets, where the cases are more or less symmetrically distributed about the mean	Mean; there should be no need to quote any other measure because all measures of central tendency for this type of data will be similar	Standard deviation and also consider giving the range
Interval, ratio or ordinal data, data heavily skewed, mean distorted by outliers	Median, though you might also quote the mean	Range and quartiles
Nominal	Mode	No measure

Having read this chapter and completed the exercises, you should be familiar with the following ideas and concepts:

- Describing data using statistics
- Measures of central tendency
- The appropriate use of the mean, median and mode
- How to calculate the mean, median and mode
- The terms 'dispersion' and 'variation'
- The appropriate use of the range, quartiles and the standard deviation
- How to calculate quartiles, the standard deviation and the variance

Exercises

1   For the study on the walk-in clinic presented in Chapter 5 calculate the mean, median and mode for the data on number of partners. (a) What is the most appropriate measure of central tendency? (b) What do these results suggest?

2   For the study on Symphadiol presented in Chapter 5 calculate the mean, median and mode for the data on the weight loss of each of the individuals in the study. (a) What is the most appropriate measure of central tendency? (b) What do these results suggest?

3   For the data in exercises 1 and 2 above, calculate the quartiles and standard deviation. Discuss which type of measure of dispersion you feel is most appropriate. What do these measures tell you about the data?

4   Find five examples where a descriptive statistic has been quoted. For each example decide whether the measure is appropriate. Discuss the measures of dispersion used with the measure of central tendency.

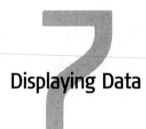

Displaying Data

Areas of learning covered in this chapter

What are the various ways of displaying data?
How to choose an appropriate way of displaying your data

This chapter will explore some of the ways that data can be displayed. It provides a rationale for the choice of display and how display type is linked with the type of data.

The two most common forms of data display are graphs and tables. Both have the same aim, to summarise and present the data in a manner that is easy to understand and take in. Displaying your data is an essential part of analysing the data. It allows you to establish how the data are distributed, to see unusual cases and generally get a 'feel' for the data.

Box 7.1

Rules

- Provide legends for tables and graphs (see p. 70).
- Categories and values must be clearly identified.
- Note units of measurement for interval/ratio data.
- Indicate total number of units.
- Identify source.

Table 7.1 Acklin and Bernat (1987) data for two indices of depression measured in patients with a range of conditions

			Patient type	
Index	LBP	Depressives	Personality disorder	Non-patients
Egocentricity	0.31	0.32	0.42	0.39
Sum morbid content	0.82	3.47	0.99	0.70

Tables present information in a text-based form. As such, much of the detail in the data can be retained. Unfortunately taking in lots of different numbers and seeing emerging patterns is rather difficult, and this is where graphs come in. When we present data in graphical form some of the detail tends to be lost but it becomes much easier to see the emerging patterns. In the example below we show some data from Acklin and Bernat (1987) in graphical (Figure 7.1) and in Table (7.1) form. Acklin and Bernat's study examined the relationship between chronic low back pain and depression. In the graph and the table we have taken two of the indices of depression that they used and plotted them against patient type.

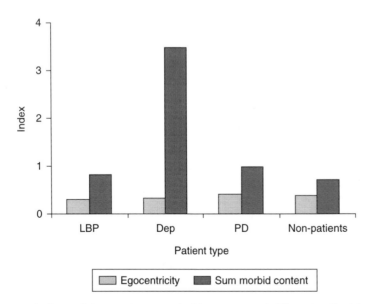

Figure 7.1   Indices of depression recorded for a range of different patient types (Acklin and Bernat 1987)

Which display form makes it easier to see the trend? Which allows you to see most detail? As a general rule the more data put into a table the more it will become harder to read, and less likely to be read. Tables should be used when the data set is very simple or when you need to show your data set in great detail. The data we used for these graphs are already summaries of the data collected. This means that the figures are averages.

Table types

There are several different types of table that can be used. Your choice of table will depend on the type and number of variables that you have. In the example above (Table 7.1) there are two types of variable. Along the top of the table we have the nominal category 'patient type' whilst down the side of the table we have two interval scale variables, that is, the indices of depression.

Table 7.2   Frequency of different ethnic groups of a sample of 178 individuals interviewed in north-east London

Ethnic group	Frequency in sample
White European (EU)	75
African	35
Indian	32
Afro-Caribbean	26
Other	10

Other tables may have just one variable which runs either along the top or down the side of the table. The measurement could be the frequency or occurrence of that particular variable. In such a case the table becomes a 'frequency table' and it is normal to have the most commonly occurring frequency at the top (see Table. 7.2).

Sometimes tables may include summary statistics (as does Table 7.1). In Table 7.3 the bottom row is a summary of the data within the table.

Tables that report on the frequency values of two nominal variables simultaneously, and that include totals, are often used to help look for associations between variables. These tables are known as **contingency tables** and are discussed in Chapter 15.

Table 7.3   Summary examination results for a group of 122 first-year student nurses

Exam paper	% (average)
1	53
2	46
3	58
4	43
Average	50

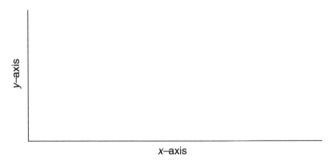

Figure 7.2   Horizontal (*x*) and vertical (*y*) axes

Graph types

The guiding principle behind using graphs is that less is more. If too much information is included in the graph the data will not be understood. All graphs are plotted against two axes, the horizontal axis and the vertical axis. The horizontal axis is known as the *x* axis and the vertical axis as the *y* axis (Figure 7.2).

An additional point to consider is that if your graph is drawn incorrectly you may mislead your audience. Figure 7.3 shows the same data twice. Both graphs indicate the average daily kcal consumption of an individual teenage girl between the ages of fourteen and eighteen. The first displays a relatively rapid increase in calorie consumption over a five-year period. In the second the increase looks much slighter. This optical illusion is caused because in Figure 7.3a the *x* axis starts at 0 but in Figure 7.3b it starts at 1,000 kcal.

Sometimes data may be presented in a manner that seeks to use graphical techniques to obscure trends rather than reveal them. Understanding graphs will help you spot this type of presentation.

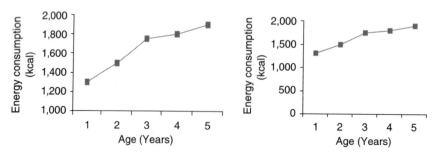

Figure 7.3　Energy consumption (kcal) in relation to age for a teenage girl between the ages of fourteen and eighteen (a) drawn with the x axis starting at 1,000 and (b) with the x axis starting at 0

Box 7.2

Axes

- Do not need to start from 0.
- Should increase in units appropriate to the measure.

There are a variety of graph types. The main types you will see are frequency charts, histograms, bar charts, pie charts, scatter graphs and line graphs. The type of chart that you should use depends on the type and complexity of the data. We will now discuss each of these in turn.

Frequency charts

We quite often divide data into categories and/or counts of how often a particular value occurred. These counts of occurrence are known as frequencies. The simplest form of data is nominal data, where we categorise things, then count the number of things in each category. Some examples of such categories are the number of males and females, different types of diseases or the number of individuals belonging to each ethnic group. To display such counts or frequencies a form of **bar chart** can be used. Figure 7.4 shows an example relating the number of visits to an eye clinic and social class.

If these data are measured initially on an interval or ratio scale, the most appropriate form of display is a **histogram**. Plotting data using a **frequency histogram** allows us to get an idea of how the data are distributed and also to get a 'feel' for the data.

In a frequency histogram, the x axis covers the range of values of the cases. Each distance covered by a 'bar' on the x axis represents a range of potential recordable values for the measure. You need to decide the size

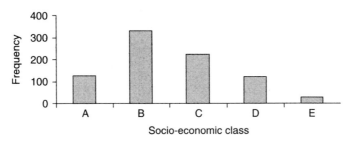

Figure 7.4 Comparison of frequency of visit to an eye clinic and socio-economic status

of the range categories that you will use. If you have too few categories the detail and patterns will be lost. If you have too many categories the patterns will be lost in the detail. Once you have decided on the range of each of your categories, you count the frequency of the number of cases in each range. Then plot a horizontal bar above the range on the x axis at the height on the graph indicated by the y axis.

The y axis displays the number of times (frequency) that a particular case value is recorded. Table 7.4 shows the peak flow rates for twenty males and twenty females. For the data for males, the range categories we have used and their associated frequencies are shown in Table 7.5.

Table 7.4 Peak Flow (l/s) measurements from twenty males and twenty females

Females	Males
563	654
605	736
631	663
618	717
623	706
657	732
585	661
600	716
574	722
604	718
612	687
622	716
670	714
604	666
612	684
577	729
596	735
684	650
698	683
594	719
Mean 616	Mean 700

Table 7.5   Ranges and frequency of peak flow measurements taken from twenty male patients

Range	Frequency
640–660	2
661–680	3
681–700	3
701–720	7
721–740	5

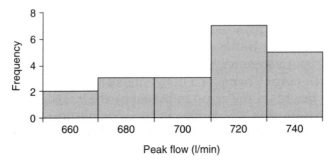

Figure 7.5   Frequency histogram of the peak flow measurements of twenty male patients

Pie Charts

Pie charts are an alternative form of frequency chart. Pie charts are best used with nominal or ordinal scale data. A pie chart displays the count of things in each nominal group category as a proportion or frequency of the total number of counts. The total data set is represented as a circle; the circle is divided into segments the size of which reflects the frequency of each nominal group. For example, Figure 7.6 shows the results

---

Box 7.3

The first?

During the Crimean War, Florence Nightingale recorded the impact of her various interventions on the morbidity of injured soldiers, using pie charts. Florence Nightingale's work probably represents one of the first uses of pie charts and of a systematic evidence-based approach to the provision of nursing care.

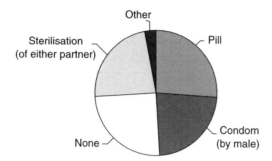

Figure 7.6   Pie chart showing choice of contraception among women aged fifteen to fifty

of a survey of the choice of contraception by women (between the ages of fifteen and fifty) carried out by the UK Department of Health in 1999.

Pie charts are ideal for simple data. If you want to divide the data further – say, for example, you were interested in the choice of contraception by different age groups within the population – then you might want to present a pie chart for each sub-group. The difficulty here is that as you start to use more pie charts it becomes more and more difficult for the eye to draw comparisons. As a rough guide, three pie charts should be the maximum. Any more and you will make it difficult for your reader. If you want to draw comparisons between different categories consider using a bar chart, as this makes it easier for the reader (see Figure 7.1).

Bar charts for summary statistical information

Bar charts can also be used to display summary statistical information such as means and standard deviations (Chapter 6). In Figure 7.1 the means of two indices of depression are plotted on a bar chart. We could

---

Box 7.4

Remember!

- Bar charts can also be incomprehensible if too many categories are used in stacked bar charts.
- For nominal and ordinal data there is always a space in between the bar to indicate that the scale of measurement is not continuous.

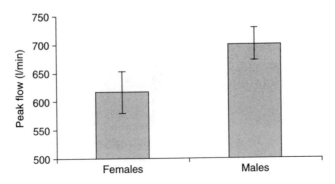

Figure 7.7   Mean peak flow for a group of twenty males and twenty females.
Horizontal bars represent ± 1 SD

also plot on the graph an indication of the variation in the data; this is often done in the form of error bars. Error bars are small vertical lines with horizontal bars at the top and bottom that mark the range of the mean plus or minus one standard deviation or standard error (see Chapter 8). For the data on peak flow, we can show the mean for each gender and give a graphical representation of the standard deviation in the form of error bars (Figure 7.7). This lets your audience see quickly how much variation there is in your samples.

Scatter graph (scatter plot)

A scatter graph is used where we are interested in whether or not there is an association between two variables, that is, is the value of one of the variables linked with the value of another? For example, weight and height are quite often closely linked. Scatter graphs can be used with interval, ratio or ordinal data that have been collected in pairs (for instance, you have measured both the height and the weight of each of your participants).

The x axis carries the scale for one of the variables, the y axis the other. Points are plotted on the graph for each sample unit. A point is plotted at the place where the values of x and y for a particular sampling unit meet. If you have sufficient data, the graph will show a scatter of points over the surface of the graph, which with a bit of luck may show a trend (Figure 7.8). You may want to fit a trend line to this type of data (see Chapter 16).

Line graphs

A line graph is similar to a scatter graph except that the points are plotted in sequence as the values increase along the x axis and a line is drawn

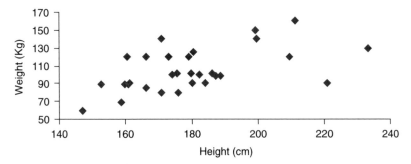

Figure 7.8   Relationship between height and weight in thirty white European males

between each point and the next. Line graphs are ideal for showing sequences, for example plots of patient observations over time, or the growth of infants over time. In general, line graphs should be used only when there is a very good reason to assume that the line drawn between the points does really represent what in all probability will happen. As such they should not really be used for grouped data, such as monthly means or counts. In practice they often are. In fact, used in this way, line graphs are quite a good way of allowing comparisons in trends across different groups of data. In Figure 7.9 the height of boys and girls is compared over time.

Presenting data is something of an art. There are some basic rules that help, outlined below and in Table 7.6. In the past it was normal to use pen and paper to produce graphs. Now it is much more common to use a computer. We have drawn all the graphs in this book using Microsoft Excel. It is worth noting that the basic unchanged (default) output from

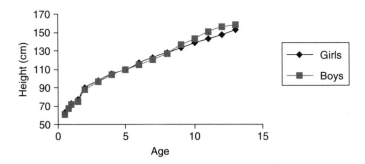

Figure 7.9   Line graph showing how average height varies with age in a sample of girls and boys

many software packages used to draw graphs is initially quite poor. You will need to work with the package to produce the output that you want.

Guidelines for drawing perfect graphs

- Keep your graph simple, with few variables. Don't select the complex option.
- Label axes and variables clearly.
- Each graph should have a legend. This is a short description of the graph and a reference to the key points and the sample size.
- Don't forget a key if there is more than one variable or group.
- Make sure you plot the points accurately. Don't use large markers.
- Choose an appropriate scale. Many computer packages will not do this for you, so you will need to practise.
- Make sure the units on the scale change in a way that suits the data.

Table 7.6   Types of graph

Type	When to use
Histogram	For showing a frequency distribution of data measured on the interval or ratio scales
Bar chart	Use for displaying frequencies of nominal or ordinal data, also for comparing measures of central tendency between groups for data measured on ordinal, interval or ratio scales
Pie chart	Used largely for showing the frequency distribution of nominal data. Try to avoid using pie charts to compare different groups of data
Scatter graph	Use with interval, ratio or ordinal data when you want to see if two variables are linked. Two or more variables must be measured from each sampling unit
Line graph	Used for data measured on interval, ratio or ordinal scales, particularly when you want to display a trend or change over time. Particularly useful for displaying trends in several groups of data at once. Avoid joining points if there is no reason to do so

Having read this chapter and completed the exercises, you should be familiar with the following ideas and concepts:

- The importance of displaying data
- How to choose an appropriate display
- Types of table
- Using tables
- Using graphs
- Selecting the appropriate graph
- Bar charts, histograms, pie charts, scatter graphs and line graphs

Exercises

1 From the questionnaire data (Chapter 5) select the most appropriate method to display the number of patients presenting (frequency) with each type of symptom.

2 From the study into Symphadiol select and display the data of the mean weight loss from each of the study groups such that a comparison can be made. Include in your display a measure of the standard deviation.

3 Take your resting pulse, then perform some light physical exercise. (Be careful if you are not particularly fit.) After the exercise, at intervals record your pulse. Repeat this five times. (Record the time interval.) Plot a graph showing the change in pulse rate with time.

4 Review three articles that use graphs to display their data. For each decide (a) if the display is appropriate, (b) if the authors followed our rules, (c) how the display could be improved.

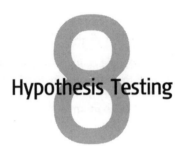

Hypothesis Testing

Hypotheses

We will now discuss the concept of hypotheses, as they are central to most studies that involve the collection of quantitative data and statistics. But what are hypotheses and, more importantly, how do they relate to the study of health? Hypotheses are essentially about prediction, which is discussed in Chapter 9. Hypotheses are central to experimental research. Strictly speaking, an experiment is an investigation where the researcher controls for some of the variables whilst manipulating others.

When we talk about a **hypothesis** we mean a method of synthesising an idea or an explanation; it is more than simply the idea or theory we are studying. The hypothesis is a proposed explanation for an observation that leads to a prediction(s) that through our investigation and the use of statistics we will

> Something to remember:
> *hypotheses* is the plural of *hypothesis*.

either confirm or reject and in so doing test the validity of the hypothesis. Hypotheses are generally built from a previous observation or experience.

In general, a hypothesis will lead to a prediction that there is a relationship or link between two or more variables. In the sexual health questionnaire described in Chapter 5 we are interested in studying the relationship between sexual activity and sexual health. In the Symphadiol trial we are interested in obesity and how it affects post-operative recovery time. Within these broad areas of study, we have some specific relationships we wish to explore.

Forming the hypothesis for the experiment/study

One of the hypotheses from the first investigation is that *males are less likely to use the walk-in clinic than females*. One of the hypotheses from the second study is that *obese patients treated with Symphadiol will lose weight faster than those not given the drug*. The predictions are highlighted in Italics.

Box 8.1

Hypothesis building

Observation A sexual health clinic manager reports that patients from certain post-code areas seem to be infrequent visitors to the clinic.

Hypothesis Individuals who live farther away from the clinic are less likely to visit.

Study Make a detailed analysis of the distance people live away from the clinic and the frequency of visits.

Experimental approaches

Some investigations will seek to test these relationships using experiments as a method of finding answers. Experiments attempt to keep the variables we are not interested in constant. This means, for example, in the second investigation we would split the patients into two groups and subject one group to treatment with Symphadiol.

We could control variables that we were not interested in, such as the patient's sex, age and socio-economic group, by carefully making sure the composition of the two groups was similar. Because we have manipulated one of the groups of people taking part in the study, this investigation is an experiment. Note that in the past people taking part in a study were known as 'subjects'. It is now becoming more common to refer to them as *participants*, in recognition that, in most cases, we must obtain consent from people before we study them and they are therefore participants in the study rather than objects to be studied.

The manipulated group is known as the **experimental or treatment** group; the group which was not subject to the manipulation is known as the **control** group. Quite often in medical studies the control group may receive a *placebo*. A placebo looks and feels to the participant like the treatment, but it has no biological activity. In statistical terms, the experimental treatment and the control groups together are known as the *treatment groups*. The results of the experiment will be subjected to statistical analysis in order to assess the likelihood of the results occurring by chance.

Non-experimental methods (sometimes called quasi-experiments)

The hypothesis from the walk-in clinic study that males are less likely to visit the walk-in clinic than females would probably not use an experiment as the basis of the investigation but a study based on the statistical analysis of data relating to the frequency of visits by males and females. This study would seek to test if the observed ratio of males to females visiting the clinic was likely to occur by chance. In this type of approach there is no control.

In non-experimental studies, rather than control variables we tend to measure all the variables we think could have an influence on the phenomenon of interest. We then try to take account for them, using statistics. For more guidance on types of quantitative research design see Depoy and Gitlin (1993).

Having read this section, you should now be aware of:

- what is meant by the term 'hypothesis'
- the difference between an experimental and a non-experimental study
- by reading chapter 2 in conjunction with chapter 8, how statistics can be used to test hypotheses

Variables

Given that we have determined that a hypothesis is a prediction concerning two or more variables, it is important to remain aware of the role of each of the variables when we apply a statistical test. For the statistical tests described in this book, we will have one **dependent variable** and at least one **independent variable**.

Dependent variable

As the name implies, the dependent variable refers to a variable whose value is determined by or dependent on the value of another variable. We may for example hypothesise that blood pressure and age are linked. If we were studying this relationship the dependent variable would be age, as we would be predicting that age in some way was important in determining blood pressure. We would not, however, suggest that age was determined by blood pressure.

Independent variable

The independent variable, on the other hand, is the one thought by the researcher to determine the value (at least in part) of the dependent variable. If we consider the relationship between blood pressure and age, we could suggest that age in some way may account for the level of blood pressure recorded. Thus age is the independent variable. For experimental designs, the independent variable is the variable that is fixed or manipulated by the person doing the experiment. If looking, for example, at the relationship between bacterial growth in culture and temperature, the experimenters control the range of temperatures they wish to use. In experimental designs the dependent variable is always the variable that is measured.

In the Symphadiol experiment described previously the independent variable is the treatment group (either Symphadiol-treated or control) the patients are assigned to the treatment groups; the dependent variable is the weight loss. Weight loss is the variable that will be measured.

In the study of visits to the sexual health clinic (Box 8.1) and distance travelled, distance travelled will be the independent variable, and the number of visits to the clinic the dependent variable. This is so because we are hypothesising that the number of visits to the sexual health clinic will depend on how close the patient lives to the clinic.

Other variables

Another important type of variable is the **confounding** variable. A confounding variable is one that has influence on the value of the dependent variable yet is not important with respect to the hypothesis that is being tested. For example, in the test of the impact of Symphadiol it could be that the *age* of the patient *influences* the effects of Symphadiol. If this is the case and we fail to ensure that both treatment groups have participants of similar age, then age will become a **confounding variable**, and the results of our experiment may be difficult to interpret. Potential confounding variables need to be taken into account using appropriate and carefully thought out research designs, particularly with respect to the selection of the sample.

Box 8.2

Short exercise

Find two research papers, on a subject that interests you, where the authors have used statistics. For each study, decide:

- What the hypothesis is.
- How many variables are being tested.
- What the independent variable(s) is.
- What the dependent variable(s) is.
- How many treatment groups there are.

Errors and statistics

In statistical terms an error is something that may give us a false result. There are several types of error. They fall into four categories: random error, sampling error, measurement error and experimental error. These are discussed at length in Chapter 3. Much of research design and statistics involves either trying to reduce error or trying to take account of it. One of the most important uses of statistics is thus to help decide if an observed result could be due to chance, that is, caused by sampling and other non-systematic errors.

Let's say that you are carrying out our second investigation. Having collected the data (Chapter 5), plotted and calculated the means, you will

Box 8.3

Chance

By 'chance' we mean something that just happens by luck or fortuitously; something without an assignable cause. 'Random' is another name for an event that is determined by chance.

see that there is a difference between the group of patients who were treated with Symphadiol and those who were not. The question facing the researcher analysing the data is: is this difference due to **chance** or is it due to the treatment? Such questions form the basis of all statistical testing.

We no longer just want to describe the data, we want to use statistics to infer things from the data and enhance the treatment and care of patients. So the important question for the researcher is: are the relationships we see down to chance? On the other hand, are they real? Errors can lead us to draw incorrect conclusions. The use of statistics will help inform us if the observed result is valid (meaning real) or if it is caused by chance.

The statistical hypothesis

The researcher establishes an experimental hypothesis before performing an experiment or study to test it. In a similar fashion, when we test the results of the experiment to see if they could have occurred by chance, we also establish a statistical hypothesis. The most common form of statistical hypothesis is the hypothesis of no difference, often called the **null hypothesis** and given the symbol H_0. The hypothesis is given the symbol H_1.

It is here that beginners at statistics often become a little confused. Take your time and practise using the exercises.

Observation

In the study of the walk-in centre, we would gather data on the frequency of visits by males and females. Having displayed these data in an appropriate manner, we notice there is a difference in the frequency of visits of males and females. This is known as the observation.

Null hypothesis

The null hypothesis for this observation is that although there appears to be a difference in the frequency of visits between males and females this observation is caused by chance and in an investigation based on the whole population there would *not* be a difference. We would now conduct a statistical test that is appropriate (that is, a test designed for the type of data that was collected). The answer to this test would give us an indication of the probability of the observation being due to chance. From this test we would either reject or accept the null hypothesis.

In the study of the effects of Symphadiol on weight loss, we would gather data on the weight loss of the groups of patients, those who were given the drug and the others who were not. Having completed the study, and plotted the data using a bar chart (see Chapter 7), you see that there is a difference between the treatment groups.

The null hypothesis for this observation is that although there appears to be a difference between the two treatment groups (that is, those in the group of participants given the drug showed greater weight loss than those who weren't), this observation is caused by chance and in an investigation based on the whole population there would *not* be a difference between the two variables. We would now conduct a statistical test that is appropriate. The answer to this test would give us an indication of the probability of the observation being due to chance. From this test we would either reject or accept the null hypothesis.

If we reject the null hypothesis we then say that the observed result is **statistically significant**. This is a very important concept and means that we have a specific degree of certainty that the observed result is real.

In research papers it is common to find that the statistical hypotheses are implied rather than stated explicitly. It is a good idea, until you become confident with statistics, to state what the null hypothesis is before conducting a statistical test.

Types of interaction between variables

When we conduct studies we are not always looking for the same type of relationship between variables. In general, there are three types of interaction: differences, relationships and associations. Deciding on the type of interaction between the variables you are dealing with is a very important aspect of statistics. This is because the type of interaction between variables will in part determine the statistical test that you use.

What is meant by difference is clear-cut. In the Symphadiol experiment we were looking to see if there was a *difference* in the weight loss between the treatment groups. If we are looking for a relationship we would be looking to see if two (or more) variables vary with each other, i.e. if you change one variable do you get a change in the other? For example, is the incidence of lung cancer related to the number of cigarettes smoked each day?

In the walk-in clinic study we were looking to see if there was an **association** between gender and frequency of visit. An association is really a special form of relationship but here we are asking the question: is one variable commonly found with a second variable? For example, we could ask the question 'Is skin cancer found more commonly (associated) in males or females?'

The problem with clinical and statistical significance

Just because you find a result isn't caused by chance (statistically significant) doesn't mean you paint the town red or even jump out of the bath shouting 'Eureka.' Now is the time for some calm thinking. Was the experiment or study conducted correctly? When research papers are published or sent for review the authors will always say the results are significant but the critics will always question whether or not the experiment was conducted correctly. Statistics cannot make up for poor experiment design.

Just because a result is statistically significant doesn't mean it is of clinical significance, in other words, that practice should be altered because of it. Let's imagine you discover that drinking ten pints of water per day reduces the incidence of acute myeloid leukemia (AML) by 10 per cent, in other words one in ten people who previously would have contracted AML will no longer do so as long as everyone drinks ten pints of water per day. However, if the incidence of contracting AML is one in 32,500, drinking ten pints of water will reduce this to just one in 35,750. Is this a sufficient drop to justify the recommendation? In health care it is also essential to take into account any side effects of proposed treatments.

Having read this chapter and completed the exercises, you should be familiar with the following ideas and words:

- Experimental and statistical hypothesis
- Control group
- Experimental treatment group
- Treatment group
- Statistically significant
- Independent, dependent and confounding variables
- Chance
- Error

Exercises

1   For the study on Symphadiol explained in Chapter 5, if you were just looking at the effect of Symphadiol (not exercise), describe: (a) the experimental hypothesis (If one exists), (b) the statistical hypothesis (H_1), (c) the null hypothesis H_0, (d) the independent variable, (e) the dependent variable.
2   For each of the experiments/studies given in Chapter 5 describe the likely source of error.

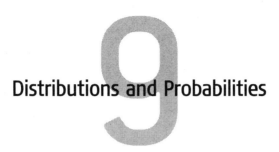

Distributions and Probabilities

Areas of learning covered in this chapter

What are	probabilities?
How are	probabilities linked with statistics and frequency distributions?
How can	frequency distributions be used to make predictions?
What types of	distributions are there?

One of the more important concepts in statistics is the idea that numbers can be distributed in certain ways. What we mean by 'distributed' is the frequency of occurrence of particular numbers. For example, a data set of the number of sexual partners that each individual has during a lifetime could contain just the values 4 or 3; it's much more likely that it will be a mixture of different numbers, from high to low. The mixture is very important, because the way your numbers are mixed or distributed will largely determine the type of statistical test that you use. The easiest way to see the way in which data combinations are assembled is to plot them in a **frequency histogram** (Figure 9.1).

Frequency histograms

The frequency histogram is really a type of bar chart where the *y* axis is the frequency of occurrence of a particular case. On the *x* axis we have

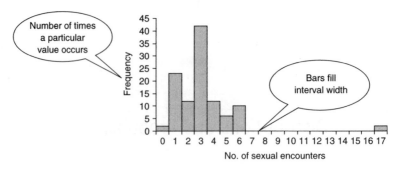

Figure 9.1   Histogram showing the frequency distribution of the number of sexual partners for 109 women aged thirty who responded to a questionnaire distributed in the London borough of Southwark

a scale that is bounded by the values of the lowest and the highest of the cases. In between are placed the values of the scale, using suitable intervals. A bar is drawn that fills the whole of each of the intervals being measured; the sides of the bars are parallel and the width of the bar is held constant.

This type of figure is normally used for variables that are recorded on an **interval** or **ratio** scale. If your data are interval or ratio scale, data plotting them in this manner must be one of your very first steps. This is because the distributions of data and

> Using the data given in Chapter 5 for the walk-in clinic, make a histogram of the number of sexual encounters reported during a three-month period.

numbers form the basis of many statistical tests. You will find that numbers are distributed in many ways. Some of the distributions have characteristics that can be exploited by researchers. One such distribution that we shall go on to explore is the **normal distribution**. This distribution forms the basis of many statistical tests, but first we need to discuss **probability**.

Probability and statistics

In Chapter 8 we introduced the notion of a statistical test and discussed the idea that statistical tests are performed because we want to know if the results we obtain are due to the experimental treatment or to chance. 'Chance' is a word that has the same meaning as the word 'probability'.

When we say, 'What is the chance of patient x catching malaria?' we could also say, 'What is the probability?' We could also say, 'What is the likelihood?" These phrases all have the same meaning: we want to know if something is likely to happen or not. Of these terms, probability is used more by statisticians. It is given the symbol P. P is normally recorded as values between zero (not possible) and 1 (certainty). The probability that you will die is 1; the probability that you will meet Florence Nightingale is 0.

Often in the media and elsewhere you will see probabilities reported as percentages. In this case, the probability that you will die would be recorded as 100 per cent and of you meeting Florence Nightingale 0 per cent.

Box 9.1

Expressing probabilities

Probabilities can be expressed as:

- A value between 0 and 1.
- A percentage.
- A fraction.

To help put probability more into context, imagine that you are walking down a busy street on a weekend with your eyes closed, then you suddenly open your eyes. The probability of seeing a man will be 0.5 or 50 per cent. The probability of seeing a woman will also be 0.5 (or half of 100 per cent).

What does this probability mean? Half the time when you open your eyes you will see a women and the other half a man. How do we get from a value of 0.5 to a more meaningful fraction? Well, 0.5 can also be written as 0.5/1 (try putting 0.5 in your calculator and dividing it by 1). 0.5/1 is the same as 1/2 (try putting 1 in your calculator and dividing it by 2). In statistics we record a probability of 1/2 as $P = 0.5$. In statistical testing we need to be at least 95 per cent certain that the result we obtained is true (that is, not caused by sampling error). In statistics, however, we normally express this probability in terms of doubt. Thus rather than say we want to be 95 per cent certain we would say that we are 5 per cent uncertain that the result is true. This 5 per cent value is normally expressed as $P = 0.05$. Remember, P stands for probability.

How are probabilities and distributions linked?

Say you have a bag of laundry with equal numbers of blue and pink towels. You cannot see into the bag. When you reach in and pull out a towel there are two possible outcomes: the towel will be pink or the towel will be blue.

Box 9.2

Practising your maths

- Express 0.45 as a fraction.
- Express 0.45 as a percentage.
- If you walked into a room that was occupied by fifty five men and forty five women, what is the probability that a woman would be the first person you encountered?
- What is 2/3 expressed as a probability?
- What is 2/5 expressed as a percentage?

Now if you pull out two towels the number of possible outcomes increases. It could be two blue towels in a row (BB) or a pink towel twice in a row (PP), or pink and then blue, or blue and then pink. In fact, we have four possible outcomes. So with just two events the number of outcomes and complexity are increasing. However, we can still predict what the probable combination of pink or blue towels might be.

If there are four outcomes (BB, PP, PB and BP) the chance of any one of these combinations occurring is 0.25 or 1/4. Two of these outcomes give you essentially the same combination of towels (PB, BP). Thus the chance of ending up with two pink towels in your hand is 1/4 and of two blue towels 1/4 and of one blue and one pink 1/2, that is, 1/4 +1/4.

Let's work through the obvious next step. You draw out three towels from your bag. The possible outcomes are PPP, BBB, PBB, BBP, PPB, BPP, BPB or PBP. There are eight of them. The probability of each outcome occurring is thus 1/8. We have four combinations: all blue, all pink, one pink and two blue, or two blue and one pink. So what is the probability of obtaining each of these combinations? Well, for PPP and BBB it is straightforward, as we have already said the probability of these outcomes is 1/8. There are three outcomes that give us one pink and two blue towels, so the probability of this combination is 1/8 +1/8 +1/8 = 3/8. There are

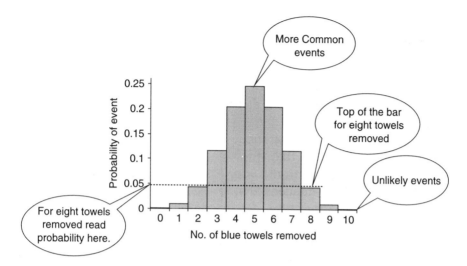

Figure 9.2   Histogram showing the probability of removing various combinations
of blue and pink towels from a bag containing of a number of blue and pink
towels in equal proportion. Remember, because ten towels were pulled out
in total, if eight blue towels are removed the other two in the set must be pink

also three outcomes that give us one blue and two pink towels, so the
probability of this combination is $1/8 + 1/8 + 1/8 = 3/8$.

You can see that as the number of events increases so the probability
of each of the outcomes changes. As the number of events increases we
need to use graphics – see Figure 9.2. It is possible to draw a histogram
that shows the probability of obtaining certain combinations, given a
certain number of events. Let's say you were pulling out ten of the towels. Now if you work through the maths you will find that here there are
eleven combinations. Using Figure 9.2, a frequency histogram, it is possible to say just how unlucky you had been if, whilst searching for ten
pink towels, you actually pulled out eight blue towels. (Find eight blue
towels on the x axis, go up to the top of the bar and read off the value
on the y axis.)

Box 9.3

Flipping a coin

If you flip a coin ten times what is the probability that a head will be turned up
just three times? – use Figure 9.2 to help.

The type of distribution shown here is called the **binomial distribution**. We have seen how it can be used to predict how rare or unusual certain events will be. This is the basis of statistical testing – asking the question 'What is the probability (likelihood) of obtaining a result by chance?' Clearly, in the example above, to pull out ten blue towels represents a rare event. We can also see that distributions of numbers and probabilities are linked.

Now the important thing about certain distributions is that they allow us to make predictions, and fortunately it just so happens that natural phenomena produce data sets that have a distribution that is similar to the one above. This distribution is known as the **normal** or **gausian** distribution. This distribution forms the basis of many of the most commonly used statistics. The type of statistics that relies on numbers being distributed in a certain way is called **parametric statistics**. We will now explore the normal distribution.

> Having read this section, you should be aware of what is meant by the term 'probability' and the ways in which probabilities can be expressed.
> You should be aware that it is possible, using a knowledge of how numbers are distributed, to make predictions.

The normal distribution curve

Imagine that the intervals on the x axis were infinitely small. Instead of a bar chart with steps we would produce a curve, particularly if we didn't shade in the bars. The normal distribution would look like such a curve (Figure 9.3). The normal distribution has mathematical properties that allow us to make predictions, just like the histogram. Note also how it is drawn, in very much the same way as Figure 9.2, as if we had connected the tops of the bars with a line and then removed the bars.

As a defined distribution curve of numbers the normal distribution has certain properties. The first is very obvious, the curve is symmetrical – you could almost say it had a certain beauty; it is sometimes referred to as 'bell-shaped'. The exact shape of the curve will depend on the standard deviation of the data. In fact it's worth remembering that the normal distribution is the construction of a mathematician's mind, so few data sets are likely to give a frequency distribution that exactly matches the normal curve.

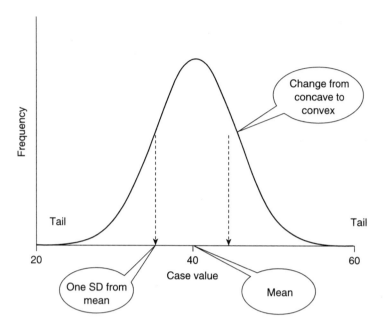

Figure 9.3   Normal distribution curve, shown here with a mean of 40 and a standard deviation of 8

The tails of a normally distributed curve (the rare values) tend to be short. Nevertheless, probably the most important feature of the normal distribution curve is that the point where the curve changes from being concave to convex (the point of inflection) is always one standard deviation (SD) away from the mean. The mean is always in the middle of the x axis. What this tells us is that the area enclosed by the boundaries of the mean plus one standard deviation and the mean minus one standard deviation is always a constant proportion of the total area, namely 68.27 per cent.

Box 9.4

The normal distribution

- is bell-shaped.
- is symmetrical.
- has short tails.
- has points of inflection that are always one standard deviation away from the mean.

In normally distributed data one standard deviation either side of the mean always encloses 68.27 per cent of the data set.

If we were to move two standard deviations away from either side of the mean then we would encapsulate 95.44 per cent of the total area. If you were to take a large sample of patients' arm lengths, you would expect that 68.27 per cent of your results would lie within ± 1 SD of the mean and that 95.44 per cent would lie within ± 2 SD of the mean.

Box 9.5

Making a prediction

You are interested in the number of Opsite dressings used on the average medical ward. You collect data from 102 wards. The data are normally distributed. How many wards will lie within ± 1 SD of the mean?
Hint: in normally distributed data 68.27 per cent of the data lie within ± 1 SD of the mean.

We have now introduced a means by which, if we know the mean and the standard deviation of a set of data, and we know that it is normally distributed, we can make predictions. We use this knowledge as the basis of what are often called **parametric statistics**.

Deviations from the normal distribution

Sometimes we find that the data we have collected do not fit the normal distribution. The best way to get a rough idea whether your data fit the distribution is to plot a frequency histogram. Some deviations have a particular shape and are given special names. The distribution shown in Figure 9.4 is called negatively skewed. This is because the mean lies to the left of the median (as you look at it). The distribution shown in Figure 9.5 is called positively skewed. This is because the mean lies to the right of the median.

Skewed data sets tend to occur when there are values which are much greater or lower than the rest. Thus the frequency histogram is not symmetrical, it's skewed. In these distributions the greater the difference between the mean and the median the greater the skew, or skewness.

It is also possible to have symmetrical distributions that do not conform to the normal distribution. The most common are random distributions and the regular, or under-dispersed, distribution. Examples of which are given below.

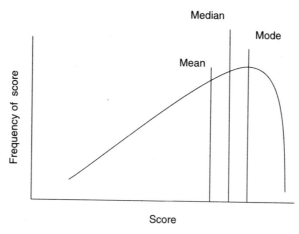

Figure 9.4   Negatively skewed distribution

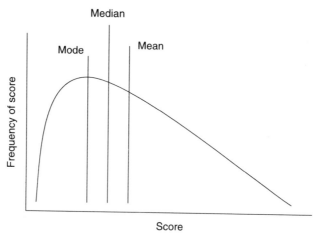

Figure 9.5   Positively skewed distribution

Random and clumped distributions

Data sets where the variance is roughly equal to the mean are referred to as *randomly distributed*. Random distribution tends to be uncommon. An example of a random distribution could be the number of occurrences of certain diseases within defined geographical areas. Such a distribution is shown in Figure 9.6 for the disease cystic fibrosis.

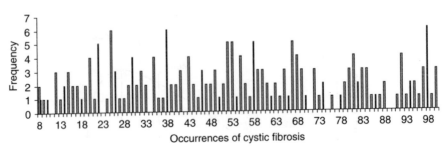

Figure 9.6   Incidence of Cystic Fibrosis in the United Kingdom, by parish.

It should be noted that true randomness is comparatively uncommon and that the geographical distribution of many disease phenomena tends to have a clumped, or over-dispersed, distribution. We talk of disease outbreaks where we recognise that particular areas have a high incidence of a certain disease. In random phenomena we are saying that each event (an occurrence of cystic fibrosis) is unrelated to any other occurrence. If the distribution is clumped it suggests that the events are related, for example in the case of a contagious disease, or a disease that is triggered by some environmental factor. Clumped distributions tend to show a strong positive skew (the mean lies to the right of the median). Such a distribution is shown for the occurrence of AIDS cases across the metropolitan districts of the United States (Figure 9.7).

The last distribution to be aware of is the **regular distribution**. The regular distribution is really an extreme form of the normal distribution. In regular distributions the standard deviation is small in relation to the

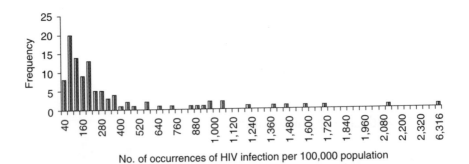

Figure 9.7   AIDS cases per 100,000 population reported in 1999, by metropolitan area. Note that the point after the value of 2,080 has a value of 6,316 and so the x-axis has been truncated. This distribution shows a strong positive skew, and so the data are clumped. The mean is 359, median 162 and the mode 47.
Source: http://www.cdc.gov/hiv/stats/hasrlink.htm

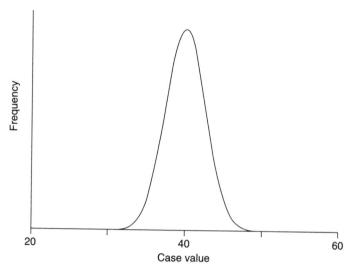

Figure 9.8   Regular distribution with a mean of 40 and a standard deviation of 2

mean, that is, there is very little spread in the data set. An example could be records of the numbers of fingers and toes within a population. Obviously, people with less than eight fingers and ten toes are unusual, and so the distribution would be regular. If a normal distribution is shaped like that shown in Figure 9.8 it is said to show **kurtosis**. It can also be said to show kurtosis if the point of the curve is flattened.

It is important to distinguish between clumped and random distributions. The manner in which data are distributed is important, as it tells us about the fundamental properties we are studying and, as we have seen here, is very relevant to studies of the distribution and spread of disease (epidemiology). We also need to know how data are distributed before we embark on many statistical tests. We can distinguish between the different types of distribution using a statistical test that will be explained later.

Having read this chapter and completed the exercises, you should be familiar with the following ideas and words:

• Frequency histogram
• Probability
• Normal distribution

Statistics for health care professionals

- Regular distribution
- Random and clumped distribution
- Skewness and Kurtosis
- The concept of a distribution of numbers and how it links with probability
- The properties of the normal distribution
- The importance of knowing how your data are distributed

Exercises

1   Collect measurements of the length of the index finger from twenty indi-viduals. Plot these data using a frequency histogram. Record the gender of your participants. Discuss your result; which distribution does your figure look like?

2   Repeat exercise 1, but this time increase your sample size. If you are working with a group of people you may want to amalgamate your results (but only if you took measurements from different participants). (a) Discuss your result; which distribution does your figure look like? (b) Has the shape of the distribution changed? What does that tell you? (c) What happens to the distribution if you separate out the male participants from the females?

3   If you tossed a coin four times what is: (a) the potential combination of outcomes? (b) the probability of each outcome? (c) the probability, if a coin is tossed four times, of obtaining three heads and one tail?

4   Plot the frequency distribution of the weight loss of two of the treatment groups from the Symphadiol experiment as they are at the end of the study. Do the distributions tell us anything?

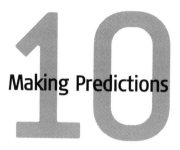

Making Predictions

This chapter begins with a little reminder. *Most health care professionals learn a lot of their art through practice. So it is with statistics, don't expect to become a practitioner of statistics without practice.*

Areas of learning covered in this chapter

How to   estimate how close a sample mean is to the population mean?
What is   the standard error?
How are   confidence limits calculated?
What are   z scores and how can they be used to make predictions?

You have seen how we can use statistics to describe data, how data can be presented as distributions of numbers and in theory how a distribution can be used to make predictions. Now we will show you how these predictions are made. We want to know, in this case, how unusual a particular event is likely to be.

The first statistic we will describe is a statistic that isn't often thought of as a prediction at all, but it most definitely is. It's also one of the most quoted statistics, and it's called the **standard error** of the sample mean (SE). So, what is it? And why is it often quoted?

The standard error of the mean provides a prediction of how close a **sample** mean is to the true **population** mean. In other words, how good was the sample? As such, it is a vital statistic. Remember, we take samples of populations normally because we don't have the resources to collect the data from the whole population. The standard error is a prediction that suggests how close our measure (taken from the sample) is to that of the true population.

Central limit theorem and standard error

The standard error relies on what at a first glance may seem rather odd but it actually makes up a 'statistical law' called the **central limit theorem**. The law basically states that if you were to collect a whole series of samples, and then plot a frequency histogram of the means of those samples, the distribution produced would be normally distributed. With the mean of that distribution (if you had collected enough random samples) being the population mean. You may want to try and prove this to yourself (see Box 10.1).

Box 10.1

Look at the sample of height measurements for the control participants from the Symphadiol experiment (Chapter 5). The mean for the sample is 179, but if you were to randomly select a sub-sample of ten cases from the control group the mean of the sub-sample would differ from 179. It would differ because of sampling error (see Chapter 3).

Take a selection of 30 sub-samples of heights from the control group and plot the means of these samples on a frequency histogram.

What shape is your histogram?

So how does the central limit theorem help us? Well, this distribution of the means of samples is normal in shape. This distribution will have the same inflected shoulders as any other normal distribution. If you remember, if we take a vertical line down to intercept the x axis, the point at which the interception occurs is normally known as the standard deviation. In the case of the distribution of sample means, it could be known as the 'standard deviation of sample means' but for simplicity we call it the **standard error**. Just as with the standard deviation, if we take the values that range from 1 SE below to 1 SE above the population mean, we will have 68.27 per cent of all the sample means. We can also predict with 68.27 per cent confidence that the population mean will be within ±1 SE of any sample mean. The standard error is simple to calculate. It is the standard deviation divided by the square root of the sample size, or:

$$SE = \frac{s}{\sqrt{n}}$$

Where s is the standard deviation and n is the sample size. When calculating the standard error by hand, find the square root of the sample size first.

The standard error of the sample mean is a prediction of how accurate a measure your sample mean is in relation to the population mean. Notice that the larger the standard deviation the larger is the standard error.

In the example from Box 10.1 you will find the mean of the control sample to be 179 with a standard error of 38.7. What this tells us is that we can be 68.27 per cent confident that the mean lies somewhere between 179 − 38.7 and

> Remember, P is shorthand for *the probability of this is* …

179 + 38.7, or between 140.3 and 217.7. Of course, what 68.27 per cent confidence means is that in only approximately sixty eight times out of 100 would this prediction be correct. In statistical terms we would say $P = 0.68$, or the probability of the population mean lying in this range is 0.68. It stands to reason, therefore, that the probability of it not being in that range is 0.32. In other words, in approximately thirty two times out of 100 the prediction would be wrong and the population mean would lie outside the predicted boundaries.

Box 10.2

Look at the data for height from the Symphadiol experiment again. Take five cases and calculate the standard error, take ten cases and calculate the standard error, finally take fifteen cases and produce another standard error.

- What does this tell you about the relationship between sample size and the standard error?
- What would happen to the standard error if the variability was lower? (Remember, we use the standard deviation as the measure of variability).
- What's the relationship between variability and the standard error?

Note that the standard error has meaning only if the data set is normally distributed. The standard error is a **parametric** statistic, that is, dependent on the distribution of the data set.

How to increase your confidence

Now, whilst you may bet £5 on a horse with odds of 68 in 100 of winning the race, it would be foolish to change a health care procedure on the basis of those odds. Really, you would like to have greater confidence in the predictions concerning health care. In practice researchers like to have 95 per cent confidence or above that the result has not occurred by chance. In some medical studies 99 per cent confidence is the accepted level. In reporting the results of statistical tests we normally report the probability of the result occurring by chance. Thus to have what is known as a **statistically significant** result, *P* (probability) must be equal to 0.05 or less, whilst in medical studies *P* must be equal to 0.01 or less.

Calculating confidence limits

This method works only for large samples where *n* is greater than 30. If we want to be 95 per cent confident in the boundaries that we predicted for the value of the population mean in relation to our estimate, all we need to do is set the boundaries to our estimate as:

$$\text{mean} \pm 1.96 \times SE$$

If we want to be 99 per cent confident we use the mean $\pm$ 2.58 $\times$ SE. Of course, we haven't plucked these values from the air, and if you want to know where they have come from you will have to read on.

Z scores

The values we used to calculate the 95 per cent and 99 per cent confidence limits are z scores from the normal distribution. Once you become more familiar with statistics, you will forget that we use z scores to give confidence limits. However, despite being a forgotten statistic, z scores can help us make predictions and plan appropriately.

So what is a z score?

A **z score** is in fact a measure of the distance along the horizontal (*x*) axis, of a frequency distribution, measured in units of standard deviation. This sounds complex but isn't really. Try to imagine it like this. Say you wanted to compare how much variation there was in lung volume among people of different countries, the only problem being that each country uses a different set of instruments to measure lung volume: some litres, some pints and some cubic feet. The first thing you would want to do is convert all the measurements to one type, a standard.

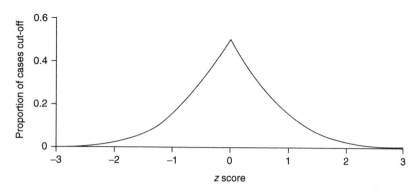

Figure 10.1   Proportion of cases cut off for a given value of *z*

In statistics it is exactly the same. If we want to measure how unusual a particular case will be we need to use a standard. We have already discussed one type of standard measurement, the standard deviation. In a normal distribution the cases that lie between + or − one standard deviation will always make up 68.27 per cent of the entire data set. What's a *z* score, then? It's the distance between the mean and any other value of interest, stated in units of standard deviation. A *z* score of 1 is equal to 1 SD. As we have said, move away from the mean in both directions, that is, + and − by one standard deviation, and you will have enclosed 68.27 per cent of all the cases in your distribution (see p. 87). If you move ±2 SD (*z* = 2) away from the mean you will enclose 95.44 per cent of all cases. As it happens ± 1.96 SD (*z* = ±) encloses 95 per cent of all cases and ± 2.58 SD (± 2.58 *z*) encloses 99 per cent. Thus a *z* score is simply a multiple of standard deviations.

For any given case, we can calculate a *z* score. You calculate a *z* score as:

$$z = \frac{\text{Case} - \text{Mean}}{\text{Standard deviation}}$$

or:

$$z = \frac{x - \bar{x}}{s}$$

OK, so what can we do with this *z* score?
Making predictions

What a *z* score can tell us is the proportion of cases that will be enclosed between the mean and that score. To find this proportion we would normally use a table of *z* scores. The table will look like Table 10.1. The first column shows z scores down to tenths of a z score. The first row shows the hundredths of a z score. For a score of 1.12 you first go to 1.1 in the first column, then across the row until you are level with 0.02 in the first row. You will need to practise calculating z scores. To be pragmatic in the following example we will use a data set of ten numbers but you need to remember that to use z scores with confidence the data set should be greater than thirty.

A nurse mentor decides she wants to compare the number of times students have given an injection during an A&E ward placement. The values are given in Table 10.2. What the nurse mentor wants to know is, what's the probability of a student nurse managing to have four opportunities or less to deliver an injection? Four is a bare minimum that the mentor wants students to achieve. So what would you need to know? Look at the equation above. To calculate z for a particular case (value) you need to enter three things (parameters) into the equation. Using the equation to calculate z:

$$z = \frac{x - \bar{x}}{s}$$

we have done the calculation:

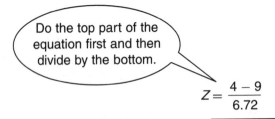

Do the top part of the equation first and then divide by the bottom.

$$Z = \frac{4 - 9}{6.72}$$

Having calculated the z score (−0.75) for the value 4, you need to look that value up in Table 10.1. This will tell you the proportion of the normal curve that is cut off at this z score. Ignore the sign. How do you

When calculating z scores the minus values tell us if the case is greater or less than. The 75 mean. −ve it's less than, +ve it's greater than.

look up this value? Go down the first column until you reach 0.7, then go across until you reach 0.05. (If you add 0.7 and 0.05 together you will get 0.75.) Read the value off the table.

OK, so with this mean and this standard deviation the proportion of the population cut off or remaining will be 0.2266, or 23 per cent. So we are predicting that the proportion of student nurses who achieve four injections or less will be 23 per cent. Clearly this chance is too high and

z	0	0.01	0.02	0.03	0.04	0.05	0.06	0.07	0.08	0.09
0	0.5000	0.4960	0.4920	0.4880	0.4840	0.4801	0.4761	0.4721	0.4681	0.4641
0.1	0.4602	0.4562	0.4522	0.4483	0.4443	0.4404	0.4364	0.4325	0.4286	0.4247
0.2	0.4207	0.4168	0.4129	0.4090	0.4052	0.4013	0.3974	0.3936	0.3897	0.3859
0.3	0.3821	0.3783	0.3745	0.3707	0.3669	0.3632	0.3594	0.3557	0.3520	0.3483
0.4	0.3446	0.3409	0.3372	0.3336	0.3300	0.3264	0.3228	0.3192	0.3156	0.3121
0.5	0.3085	0.3050	0.3015	0.2981	0.2946	0.2912	0.2877	0.2843	0.2810	0.2776
0.6	0.2743	0.2709	0.2676	0.2643	0.2611	0.2578	0.2546	0.2514	0.2483	0.2451
0.7	0.2420	0.2389	0.2358	0.2327	0.2296	0.2266	0.2236	0.2206	0.2177	0.2148
0.8	0.2119	0.2090	0.2061	0.2033	0.2005	0.1977	0.1949	0.1922	0.1894	0.1867
0.9	0.1841	0.1814	0.1788	0.1762	0.1736	0.1711	0.1685	0.1660	0.1635	0.1611
1.0	0.1587	0.1562	0.1539	0.1515	0.1492	0.1469	0.1446	0.1423	0.1401	0.1379
1.1	0.1357	0.1335	0.1314	0.1292	0.1271	0.1251	0.1230	0.1210	0.1190	0.1170
1.2	0.1151	0.1131	0.1112	0.1093	0.1075	0.1056	0.1038	0.1020	0.1003	0.0985
1.3	0.0968	0.0951	0.0934	0.0918	0.0901	0.0885	0.0869	0.0853	0.0838	0.0823
1.4	0.0808	0.0793	0.0778	0.0764	0.0749	0.0735	0.0721	0.0708	0.0694	0.0681
1.5	0.0668	0.0655	0.0643	0.0630	0.0618	0.0606	0.0594	0.0582	0.0571	0.0559
1.6	0.0548	0.0537	0.0526	0.0516	0.0505	0.0495	0.0485	0.0475	0.0465	0.0455
1.7	0.0446	0.0436	0.0427	0.0418	0.0409	0.0401	0.0392	0.0384	0.0375	0.0367
1.8	0.0359	0.0351	0.0344	0.0336	0.0329	0.0322	0.0314	0.0307	0.0301	0.0294
1.9	0.0287	0.0281	0.0274	0.0268	0.0262	0.0256	0.0250	0.0244	0.0239	0.0233
2.0	0.0228	0.0222	0.0217	0.0212	0.0207	0.0202	0.0197	0.0192	0.0188	0.0183
2.1	0.0179	0.0174	0.0170	0.0166	0.0162	0.0158	0.0154	0.0150	0.0146	0.0143
2.2	0.0139	0.0136	0.0132	0.0129	0.0125	0.0122	0.0119	0.0116	0.0113	0.0110

(Continued)

Table 10.1 (Continued)

z	0	0.01	0.02	0.03	0.04	0.05	0.06	0.07	0.08	0.09
2.3	0.0107	0.0104	0.0102	0.0099	0.0096	0.0094	0.0091	0.0089	0.0087	0.0084
2.4	0.0082	0.0080	0.0078	0.0075	0.0073	0.0071	0.0069	0.0068	0.0066	0.0064
2.5	0.0062	0.0060	0.0059	0.0057	0.0055	0.0054	0.0052	0.0051	0.0049	0.0048
2.6	0.0047	0.0045	0.0044	0.0043	0.0041	0.0040	0.0039	0.0038	0.0037	0.0036
2.7	0.0035	0.0034	0.0033	0.0032	0.0031	0.0030	0.0029	0.0028	0.0027	0.0026
2.8	0.0026	0.0025	0.0024	0.0023	0.0023	0.0022	0.0021	0.0021	0.0020	0.0019
2.9	0.0019	0.0018	0.0018	0.0017	0.0016	0.0016	0.0015	0.0015	0.0014	0.0014
3.0	0.0013	0.0013	0.0013	0.0012	0.0012	0.0011	0.0011	0.0010	0.0010	0.0010
3.1	0.0010	0.0009	0.0009	0.0009	0.0008	0.0008	0.0008	0.0008	0.0007	0.0007
3.2	0.0007	0.0007	0.0006	0.0006	0.0006	0.0006	0.0006	0.0005	0.0005	0.0005
3.3	0.0005	0.0005	0.0005	0.0004	0.0004	0.0004	0.0004	0.0004	0.0004	0.0003
3.4	0.0003	0.0003	0.0003	0.0003	0.0003	0.0003	0.0003	0.0003	0.0003	0.0002

Table 10.2   Number of injections delivered by a group of student nurses on an A&E ward

Student nurse	1	2	3	4	5	6	7	8	9	10
No. of injections	9	3	19	5	7	8	23	5	3	8

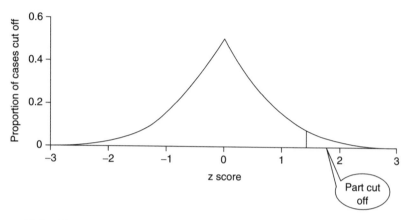

Figure 10.2   The proportion of the cases cut off at a z score of 1.3

the nurse mentor needs to rethink how this aspect of learning opportunity on the A&E placement needs to be managed.

Clearly, with a sample of ten it is relatively easy to see what the data are suggesting, without needing to calculate a z score, but say we had fifty students or even 750 to manage? Note two things here about using z scores:

- To make a prediction about a case in a distribution you need to know only the standard deviation and the mean.
- In the example above, see how close our prediction of 23 per cent is to the value that you would have guessed at (probably 20 per cent). These ten numbers are not normally distributed. (We just used them for an example.) Nevertheless, despite that, the prediction is quite close to reality. This demonstrates an important feature of tests based on the normal distribution: they tend to be what statisticians call **robust**. That is, you can break some of the assumptions and they will still work.

Another useful aspect of z scores is that they can be used in reverse, that is, say we had a set of data and we wanted to predict the value of a case that would occur at a certain probability or risk level. We will use an example to illustrate this.

Staff Nurse Andrew Peters has responsibility for maintaining clean utility supplies in a busy A&E department. He has been informed that the unit has to move to a new building. Inevitably, as with most new buildings, there is less space for storage and Andrew is concerned about the number of sterile dressings that he should stock. Fluctuating demands are placed on A&E departments and so it is difficult to predict just how many sterile dressings may be required during any particular week. Obviously, Andrew could keep a vast stock of dressings but he would have little room for anything else. Clearly he needs to make a risk assessment. The cost of overstock is wasted space, the cost of understocking may affect the ability of the department to provide appropriate care for patients.

Fortunately, Andrew has collected information on the number of dressings used per week over the last year. His sample size is thus fifty two, and he has calculated that the mean number of dressings used per week is fifty eight, with a standard deviation of nine. The theoretical normal distribution for this standard deviation and mean is shown in Figure 10.3. Now let's say that Andrew wants to be prepared for all but the most extreme circumstances. Say he decides he wants to be prepared for 99 per cent of all demand levels. He would then look in the z table for the value of 1 per cent, or 0.01 Remember, the z table tells us what's left. He must look *in* the table, *not* at the z scores down the sides. The z score is about 2.29. Now you need to do some maths. We want to know what case this z score gives us, i.e. how many dressings.

To do this we need to put the values we know into the equation we used to calculate z. Remember that s is the symbol given to the standard deviation.

$$z = \frac{x - \bar{x}}{s}$$

In Andrew's example

$$2.29 = \frac{x - 58}{9}$$

Andrew must solve the equation for the case value x. To do this, multiply both sides of the equation by 9. This gives you $20.61 = x - 58$, because you can cancel the 9s on the right-hand side of the equation. Then simply take the -58 to the other side of the equation, where it will become a $+58$, thus we have:

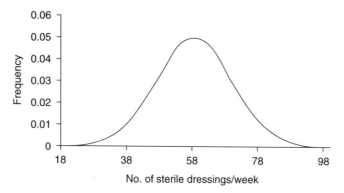

Figure 10.3   Theoretical normal distribution for a mean of 58 and standard deviation of 9

$$78.61 = x$$

Thus if Andrew wants a 99 per cent chance of never running out of sterile dressings he needs to keep about seventy nine in stock.

Having read this chapter and completed the exercises, you should be familiar with the following ideas and concepts:

- Statistics can be made to make predictions
- The standard error and confidence intervals are predictions
- How to calculate standard errors and confidence intervals of sample means
- What the term 'robust' means
- How to calculate z scores
- How to use z scores to make predictions
- That the standard error and confidence intervals predict how close a sample mean is to a population mean
- Be aware of the central limit theorem

Exercises

1   In the Symphadiol experiment the mean of the heights in the control group is 179 cm. Calculate the standard deviation, the standard error and the 95 per cent confidence limits of the mean.

2   For each of the calculations in question 1 describe what each statistic is telling you.

3 Bernard Smith is a community nurse working with a needle exchange
   programme. There is concern that the mobile unit occasionally runs out
   of clean needles. Bernard has recorded how many clean needles are
   used each night; he has calculated the mean to be seventy six and the
   standard deviation to be twenty. (a) What health care problems do you
   think running out of needles might create? (b) How might running out of
   needles undermine the programme? (c) Calculate how many needles
   Bernard needs to stock in order to be (i) 95 per cent and (ii) 65 per cent
   certain of not running out of needles.

11

Testing for Differences between Means

Areas of learning covered in this chapter

How do   I test to see if there is a difference between means?
What are   the F, z and t tests?
When   should F, z and t tests be used?
What is   the difference between a one and two-tailed test?

We have seen how we can use statistics to make predictions. Now we are going to see how we can use them to predict if the differences between two sets of results could have occurred by chance.

Box 11.1

Good design

What steps would you take to ensure that your control group was representative?

Let's say that you have set up your study, you have a control and an experimental group; the experimental group is subject to an intervention. You have been measuring patients' post-operative recovery rates on surgical wards in relation to having new therapy. In this therapy patients are played tapes of their favourite music whilst undergoing surgery. In

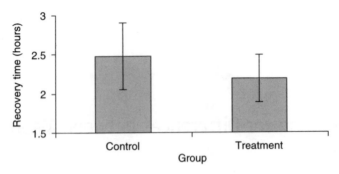

Figure 11.1   Mean post-operative recovery time of two groups of patients. The treatment group were played tapes of their favourite music

this study the variable being measured is the time taken to recover. Thus our dependent variable is time. The independent variable will be the treatment group. Patients may have been ascribed to either the study group or the control group.

Having collected your data, the first thing you should do is plot the data. This will allow you to get a handle on what your data feel like. You may want to plot the data as frequency histograms and also as bar charts, with bars showing the variation. Bars normally show either the range or the standard error, or the standard deviation. Sometimes more than one statistic is shown (see Chapter 7). You've now plotted the data. You notice that the treatment group has a faster recovery time. You will also notice by plotting a histogram if there are any unusual results (outliers).

Box 11.2

When do you need a test?

Based on the descriptives, when might you decide not to do a statistical test?

OK, so there is a difference between the mean recovery time of the two groups. The question we need to ask is how likely it is that the difference has occurred by chance, that is, is it likely that the difference is simply due to sampling errors (Chapter 8)? Remember, the data you used in Box 10.1. Those data were all drawn from the same population but the differences between the means were all different. The difference was due to sampling error. The question we are asking when we are testing to see if the observed result is probably due to chance is: do these means come from the same population (in which case there would be no difference between the population means) or do they come from two separate populations, the difference between the populations being the impact of the treatment?

The *F* test

There are a whole group of tests associated with this problem. In this chapter we will look at statistics called *F*, student's *t* and *z*. Like most statistical tests they all have rules about when they should and should not be used. In fact the art of applying statistics is to know when to use a particular test, that is, which rules apply to which. You could liken this to some therapies. For example, as practitioners you may not understand fully how a particular drug works, but based on a set of symptoms you know when to apply it and when not to. So it is with statistics. We need to know which to apply and when, and even if we don't follow the maths we can select the correct test from a computer package.

Box 11.3

Exploring the tests

Look through a few quantitative research papers that you have access to. Which statistics are used most often?

The rules for the *F*, *z* and *t* tests are the following:

- The dependent variable must be measured on the interval or ratio scale;
- The samples must come from a normally distributed population;
- With respect to *z* and *t*, the **variance** of the samples must be equal. (As you become more knowledgeable you will find there are ways around this problem.)

We will look at the variance first, as it is the basis of the *F* test. The variance is just another measure of variation; in fact, it is simply the standard deviation squared (s^2). It is used in a large number of statistical tests.

The *F* test, or, to give its full name, the **F test for equality of variance**, tests to see if the variances of the two samples are equal, or, as we

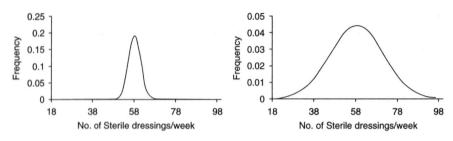

Figure 11.2   These two samples clearly differ greatly in their distribution

should say, 'not significantly different'. Why is this important? If the variances are different, it tells us that the shapes of the normal distributions that the populations are drawn upon differ markedly. If the shapes are very different it is unlikely that the mean of one sample is drawn from the same sample as the other. The shape of the distributions is as important as the means.

As you can see (Figure 11.2), the shapes of these two distributions look different. If the shapes are actually

> The symbol for the variance is s^2

statistically different there is little point in testing to see if the means come from the same population because quite clearly they do not. Thus it is good practice to apply an F test first before testing to see if there is a significant difference between the means.

The F test statistic is calculated as

$$F = \frac{\text{Greater variance}}{\text{Lesser variance}}$$

If the shape of the two distributions of the samples is identical, then F will equal 1. The greater the difference between them the larger F will be. But how do we know when to say that F is so big that the difference between them is **significant**? This comes back to the idea of probability. First we need to decide what level of probability we are working at. We said previously (Chapter 9) that it's normal to work at $P = 0.05$, that is, if the chance of getting a certain value of F is as extreme as 5 per cent (one in twenty) we say the result is significant. With this F test (known as the F test for equality of variance) we work at the 0.01 level (1 per cent, or one in 100).

If the chance of the particular value of F is *greater* than 0.01 we say that the two distributions are *not* significantly different and we should carry on to do either the z test or the student's t test. If the chance is *less* than 0.01 we say they are significantly different. The chance of obtaining a particular value of F will depend on the sizes of the samples.

Box 11.4

Record the forearm length of a group of males and a group of females.

- For each group, compute the mean, standard deviation and variance.
- Compute the F statistic for equality of variance
- State the null and alternative hypotheses.

For example, Ungamba Maliba, a mental health practitioner, is conducting some research into the impact of the drug Mindrenew (a fictitious name) on the recall speed of patients with mild Alzheimer's disease. He measures the mean ($\bar{x}$) response of the control group as 180 seconds and the standard deviation as thirty-two seconds. The mean of the treatment group is 180 seconds and the standard deviation sixty-three. Thirty-two participants took part in each group. Is there an effect of the treatment? Do the samples represent the difference or are they from the same population?

First, you would do the F test:

$$F = \frac{\text{Greater variance}}{\text{Lesser variance}} = \frac{3,969}{1,024} \quad F = 3.87$$

Having found the value of F, you must now compare it with the value in the F table, at the 0.01 level of probability (see Appendix 2). Looking at this table, notice that the top row is labelled v_1 and that first column is labelled v_2. These refer to the sample size of each of the two samples -1. In other words:

> If you use a statistical computer package, for most tests the computer will look up the value and compare it with the test statistic for you.

$$v_1 = 32 - 1 = 31$$
$$v_2 = 32 - 1 = 31$$

Now find the column in the table that starts with a value close to 31 and the row where the value is also close to 31. Note the value where these columns and rows cross. The value you should find is about 2.36.

> What could Ungamba Maliba conclude about the impact of Mindrenew on Alzheimer's disease?

Because our calculated value is *greater* than this value we can say that there is a **statistically significant difference** in the shape of the two distributions and therefore they are likely to be samples from two different populations.

Note a good rule of thumb here. When we compare the value given by a statistical test to that in a table, in general, if the calculated value is *larger than* the value in the table the result *is* statistically significant.

If we find that the result is not statistically different, we say there is *no significant difference*. This means that whilst the actual recorded values may be diffferent the high probability is that this difference has occurred by chance.

Testing for difference between the means (*z* and *t* tests)

The *z* test

Let's say that in a study the *F* test came up with the answer that there was no statistically significant difference between the two samples. You would then need to go on to test for difference between the means. The *z* test is not a test you will see quoted very often, as most researchers incorrectly opt for the *t* test. This is partly because most computer packages do not carry a facility for doing the *z* test and also any error is unlikely to affect the conclusion of the test. The *z* test should be used if your sample sizes are large, and when you are comparing the means of two samples.

If the null hypothesis (no difference) is correct, then, as we said before, any difference between the mean is simply due to sampling error. But how big does the difference need to be before we can say that they are significantly different? To answer this question we turn to *z* scores again. If the difference is greater than a *z* of 1.96 it is significantly different at the 5 per cent level (2.58 at the 1 per cent level).

But which *z*? Both distributions may have different standard deviations. The answer is that the *z* here refers to the **standard error of the difference** between the two means.

To use statistics you do not need to know how the test works, just which one to use when; but understanding a procedure will help your development as a practitioner. We include the next section just to show how the test works.

Look back at the data shown in Figure 11.1. Let's say they are from the same population, that is, the treatment had no effect. There should ideally be no difference between the means, but we know that because of error the ideal is unlikely.

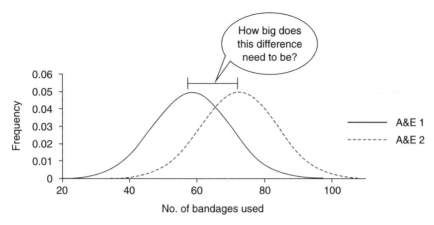

Figure 11.3   Distributions of data recording the number of bandages used on two A&E departments. The numbers clearly differ, but is the difference statistically significant?

Imagine that you drew two more samples from the population. There would again be a difference. We record this difference and then repeat again and again. We would generate a sample of differences, differences between samples. If we were to plot this sample of differences as a frequency histogram we would find, perhaps to our surprise, that it was normally distributed, with a population mean of 0. Of course, like other normal distributions, this distribution of differences has a standard deviation. This standard deviation is called the standard error of the difference.

The z test statistic asks: is the difference between the two sample means greater than the standard error of the difference? If so, how big is it? The statistic z is calculated as the difference between the sample means minus the population mean. (The population mean of this sample of differences will always be 0 if the two samples are in reality drawn from the same population.)

Box 11.5

- Using your data collected for the exercise in Box 11.4, perform a z test.
- What is the null hypothesis? What is the alternative hypothesis?
- What do you conclude?

The difference in the means is then divided by the standard error of the difference. In this case the mathematical formula does look simpler than the words:

$$z = \frac{(\bar{x}_1 - \bar{x}_2) - 0}{\text{Standard error of the difference}}$$

where is $\bar{x}_1$ the mean of sample 1 and $\bar{x}_2$ the mean of sample 2. It doesn't matter which sample you decide is to be sample 1 and which sample 2.

What we haven't told you yet is how to find the standard error of the difference. Obviously, as you have only two samples to work with, it would be difficult to produce a frequency distribution. So we have to estimate the value on the basis of the variance of the two samples. The formula to calculate the standard error of the difference is:

$$\text{Standard error of difference} = \sqrt{\frac{s_1^2}{n_1} + \frac{s_2^2}{n_2}}$$

where s is the standard deviation.

Given that you can now calculate the standard error of the difference, you can use equation 1 to calculate z. If a value you calculate is greater than 1.96 you can say that the means are significantly different at the $P < 0.05$ (5 per cent) level. If the value is greater than 2.58 you can say that the means are significantly different at the $P < 0.01$ (1 per cent) level. ($<$ is the symbol for 'less than'.) Here we have introduced the idea of different levels of significance. The levels we normally talk of are $P < 0.05$, $P < 0.01$, $P < 0.001$ and $P < 0.0001$. The lower the level of P the greater confidence you have in your result not having occurred by chance. These levels are arbitrary and it is becoming, with the advent of computers, common to quote the exact P value given by the computer package.

When we say there is a significant difference we are *rejecting* the null hypothesis. This is because the chance of getting a result (a z value) as high as this is very low.

Box 11.6

Reminder

Remember, your first steps would be to plot out your raw data and check that they were normally distributed. You would then plot the means on a bar chart, showing the extent of the variation using error bars. Then you would perform an F test. If the F test indicates that the sample sizes are not significantly different you should proceed with a test that looks at the means. As the sample size is large here, we opt for the z test.

Table 11.1   Mean results and descriptive statistics from a study on the impact of shift pattern on back injuries

Sample	No. of reported back injuries Mean ($\bar{x}$)	Standard deviation(s)	Sample size (n)
Control	21	6	182
Treatment	18	5	196

An example

Occupational health officers Smith and Meadson have been asked by their occupational health department to investigate if a new shift pattern results in more or fewer incidents of back injury. Smith and Meadson have decided to use a controlled study, and half the work force operate the old shift pattern (control group) whilst the other half operate the new system (experimental or treatment group). They measure the reported back pain per week in the two groups. The dependent variable is thus change in back pain per week. The independent variable is the experimental groups (control, and treatment). The results are shown in Table 11.1.

Step 1. Calculate the standard error of the difference:

$$\text{Standard error of difference} = \sqrt{\frac{s_1^2}{n_1} + \frac{s_2^2}{n_2}} = \cdot\sqrt{\frac{6_1^2}{182_1} + \frac{5_2^2}{196_2}} = \cdot\sqrt{\frac{36}{182_1} + \frac{25}{196_2}}$$

$$= \sqrt{\frac{61}{378}} = \sqrt{0.16} = 0.40$$

Step 2. Calculate the difference between the means:

$$\text{Standard error of difference} = (\bar{x}_1 - \bar{x}_2) - 0 = (21-18)-0 = 3$$

Step 3. Calculate z, that is, divide the result from step 2 by that from step 1.

$$z = \frac{3}{0.40} = 7.5$$

As z is bigger than both 1.96 and 2.54 we can reject the null hypothesis (no difference) and say that the means *are* significantly different and conclude that the introduction of the new shift pattern reduces the reported incidence of back pain.

Note that, having come to the statistical conclusion, that is, whether the difference is significant or not, we can move to the conclusion of the study, was the treatment effective. You decide.

The student's t test

This test should appear in all introductory tests on statistics and is still probably one of the most used tests. It is particularly of use for small-scale studies where the questions being asked are simple and the sample size is low.

With small samples it becomes difficult to make a reliable judgement or test of whether or not the samples are normally distributed. The t test makes the assumption that the parent population from which the samples are drawn is normally distri-buted. It also assumes that variances of the two samples are similar and that the data are measured on the interval/ratio scale.

> The person who invents a test often names it. The person who invented the student's t test was prevented by his employer from giving it his own name, so he called it the student's.

The t test assumes that the samples themselves are not distributed nor-mally but distributed according to the t distribution. This distribution is like a flattened normal distribution with long tails. It uses a new statistic called the pooled variance. The pooled variance is used to calculate the standard error of the difference as used in the z test. We won't go in to the theory but we will show you how the t test is carried out.

> Most computer packages do not have a facility to conduct a z test. Use a t test instead. The result will be equivalent.

The pooled variance is calculated as:

$$s_c^2 = \frac{n_1 s_1^2 + n_2 s_2^2}{n_1 + n_2 - 2}$$

Here S_c^2 is the pooled variance, n_1 is the sample size for sample 1, n_2 is the sample size for sample 2, S_1^2 is the variance for sample 1 and S_2^2 is the variance for sample 2. t itself is given by the equation:

$$t = \frac{(\bar{X}_1 - \bar{X}_2) - 0}{S_c \times \sqrt{\frac{1}{n_1} + \frac{1}{n_2}}}$$

Box 11.7

- Using your data collected for the exercise in Box 11.4, perform a t test.
- What is the null hypothesis? What is the alternate hypothesis?
- What do you conclude?
- Is a z test or a t test more appropriate?

Table 11.2 Mean results and descriptive statistics from a study on the impact of a new manipulation on recovery from knee surgery

Sample	Angle of contraction mean ($\bar{x}$)	Standard deviation(s)	Sample size (n)
Control	11.2	3.12	14
Treatment	10.3	2.54	14

Here S_c is the square root of S_c^2. The rest of the symbols you have met before.

An example

Mary Smith is a physiotherapist who is working as part of a multi-professional health care team who treat osteoarthritis. She is interested in evaluating the effect of a new manipulation therapy regime on the recovery of patients who have had surgery to insert artificial knee joints.

She has obtained consent from the ethics committee to conduct her research, and sixty patients have volunteered. Unfortunately only twenty-eight of these patients are within the exact **target group** that the team is interested in (for example, correct age and sex). Fourteen patients are allocated to the treatment group and fourteen to the control group.

As a measure of recovery Mary Smith has chosen to use the angle of contraction that patients are able to achieve without pain when moving from a standing to a crouching position. The dependent variable is thus the angle. The independent variable is the experimental group, either control or treatment.

As with the z test, having collected the data, the first steps would be to plot the data, then to conduct an F test. If the F test indicates that the variance is similar (not significantly different) you would proceed with the t test. We use a t test here because the sample size is small, and we have a good idea that the parent population would be normally distributed.

> S^2 (the variance) is the standard deviation squared.

Step 1. Calculate the pooled variance:

$$S_c^2 = \frac{n_1 s_1^2 + n_2 s_2^2}{n_1 + n_2 - 2}$$

$$= \frac{14 \times 3.12^2 + 14 \times 2.54^2}{14 + 14 - 2} = \frac{14 \times 9.73 + 14 \times 6.45}{26}$$

$$= \frac{136.22 + 90.3}{26} = \frac{136.22 + 90.3}{26} = \frac{226.52}{26} = 8.71$$

Step 2. Calculate t (remember to convert S_c^2 to S_c):

$$t = \frac{(\bar{x}_1 - \bar{x}_2) - 0}{S_c \times \sqrt{\frac{1}{n_1} + \frac{1}{n_2}}}$$

$$t = \frac{11.2 - 10.3}{2.95 \times \sqrt{\frac{1}{14} + \frac{1}{14}}} = \frac{0.9}{2.95 \times \sqrt{0.071 + 0.071}} = \frac{0.9}{2.95 \times 0.142}$$

$$= \frac{0.9}{0.419} = 2.15$$

So $t = 2.15$. You now need to look this value up in the t distribution tables, using the sample size of twenty-eight. However, when using a t test and many other tests, rather than use the actual sample size we use something called the degrees of freedom. In the case of the student's t test the **degrees of freedom** are the total sample size -2 (because there are two experimental groups). So we have $28 - 2$ degrees of freedom, or twenty-six. If you go to Table 3 in Appendix 2 you will see degrees of freedom, or d.f., down the first column and significance levels across the top.

Mary Smith is conducting a clinical study and therefore feels it is appropriate to work at the 0.01 (1 per cent) level. Look down the 0.01 column until it meets the row for twenty-six degrees of freedom. The value is 2.779. Our calculated value is much smaller than this. As our value is smaller than that in the table, we can say that there is *no* statistically significant difference. Mary Smith can therefore conclude that the new therapy regime does not result in a significant improvement in the recovery of her patients with respect to the measured variable at the time of testing.

Box 11.8

Expressing the results

When you describe the results of a statistical test you must tell the reader the type of test used, the value of the test statistic, the sample size, and at what probability level the result was significant (or not). In Mary Smith's study we would say there was no statistically significant difference between the control and the treatment group (student's $t = 2.78$, $n = 28$, $P > 0.01$).

If you look at the t test you will see that although the maths is not that complex a number of calculations are involved. You will also realise that performing all these calculations by hand is laborious and prone to error, hence the evolution of the statistical computer package. We would recommend that you use a computer package whenever one is available.

Power

We have said that the t test is designed for small sample sizes, but how small? You can perform the calculations on very small samples, but in practice as

> Contrast the term *Power* with the term *Robust*

your sample size becomes smaller your tests will tend to give the outcome of 'no significant difference' more often, even if in reality your treatment has an effect. This is because as your sample size becomes smaller the **power** of the statistical test becomes less. Power in statistical terms means the *ability to show a statistically significant result* if there is indeed one.

Paired t test

Another type of t test you will come across is called the paired t test. This test is a member of a type of test known as **repeat measures designs**. The tests we have described so far all involve situations where we have allocated participants to one group or another (control or treatment). What if we want to see the impact of a treatment before and then after an intervention? This would be an example of a repeat measures design because we would repeat the measurements on the same participants.

When we do this type of study we actually have less error to contend with, because using the same participants removes all the error associated with using two different groups of people, that is, we no longer need to take into account the natural variation in response that occurs between the participants, and we can focus on the difference before and after. The maths of the test is slightly different but the principle is identical. Again the variables must be measured using the interval/ratio scale.

Example

Mohammed Dhauba, a consultant nurse in a cardiac out-patients' unit, is concerned that most of his patients' diastolic blood pressure is higher on initial measurement than on subsequent measurement. The difference could be for several reasons. He decides to investigate whether or

Table 11.3 **Mean results and descriptive statistics from a study on the difference between initial and subsequent measures of diastolic blood pressure**

Sample	Mean ($\bar{x}$) diastolic blood pressure (mm Hg)	Standard deviation(s)	Sample size (n)
10 Minutes.	94.23	10.17	20
2 hours	85.58	8.19	20

not it is true and to determine the significance of his findings for his patients.

He measures the blood pressure of twenty patients within ten minutes of them entering the out-patients' department and then *repeats* the measurement two hours later. Because Mohammed repeats the measurement on the same participants, he knows he needs to use a repeat measures design test. Because he has two experimental groups (after ten minutes and then two hours later) and his sample is rather small he selects a paired t test. Here the **dependent variable** is blood pressure and the **independent variable** is time. The summary statistics are shown in Table 11.3

The mechanics of the paired t test retreats back to using the standard error of the difference, as in the z test. Obviously, if you are measuring the same person, if there is no effect of the time interval then the difference between the measurements will be 0. Thus the mean of all the participants' differences will be 0 if there is no effect. However, because of error we know it's unlikely that even if the treatment has no effect the means will equal 0. But how big does that deviation need to be? This is exactly the same question that we posed with respect to the z test and the answer is the same, the only difference being that we can actually calculate the mean of the differences and calculate the standard error of these differences.

> In the paired t test it is the differences that need to be normally or assumed to be normally distributed, not the measurement variables themselves.

The formula for the paired t test is:

$$t = \frac{\Sigma d}{\sqrt{\frac{n\Sigma d^2 - (\Sigma d)^2}{n-1}}}$$

Again, a complex-looking formula but taken step by step it is really not that bad. Here d refers to the difference between the initial measurement

Table 11.4 The differences between initial measures of diastolic blood pressure and those taken ten minutes later

Individual participant	Blood pressure after 10 minutes mm Hg	Blood pressure after two hours mm Hg	d	d²
1	109	88	+21	441
2	104	84	+20	400
3	84	86	-2	4
4	80	84	-4	16
5	90	75	+15	225
6	107	81	+26	676
7	106	92	+14	196
8	98	86	+12	144
9	78	90	-12	144
10	89	82	+7	49
11	91	77	+14	196
12	85	95	-10	100
13	87	88	-1	1
14	101	84	+17	289
15	94	88	+6	36
16	87	75	+12	144
17	85	94	-9	81
18	111	73	+38	1444
19	103	82	+21	441
20	97	107	-10	100
			$\Sigma d = 175$	$\Sigma d^2 = 5127$

for an individual and the subsequent one. The symbol Σ (an upper-case sigma) means 'the sum of'; you met it in Chapter 6 on descriptive statistics. Σd means all the differences between the two measurements of the individuals added together. To do this test by hand you need all the raw data.

When doing a paired test there is no need to test for equality of the variance.

Step 1. Prepare a table of results and calculate Σd and Σd^2.
Step 2. Calculate $(\Sigma d)^2$, in this case 175^2, which equals 30,625.
Step 3. Feed the values into the equation:

$$t = \frac{\Sigma d}{\sqrt{\dfrac{n\Sigma d^2 - (\Sigma d)^2}{n-1}}} = \frac{175}{\sqrt{\dfrac{(20 \times 5,127) - 30,625}{20-1}}}$$

$$= \frac{175}{\sqrt{\dfrac{102,540 - 30,625}{19}}} = \frac{175}{\sqrt{\dfrac{102,540 - 30,625}{19}}}$$

$$= \frac{175}{\sqrt{3,595.75}} = \frac{175}{59.96} = 2.91$$

Look up your value of *t* in Appendix 2, Table 3, using the appropriate number of degrees of freedom, in this case d.f. = 19.

The degrees of freedom used in this test equal *n*–1. The value of *n* in the paired *t* test, as in all statistical tests, is the sample size. You may be thinking 'but I have made forty measurements.' However, because the test works on the difference between the two measures on the same subject, you actually have only twenty samples of differences so n = 20 and d.f. 19.

So you look up 2.91 in the table for nineteen degrees of freedom. The figure 2.91 is greater than the value of 2.093 for the *P* = 0.05 level of significance and also for that of 2.861 for the *P* = 0.01 level. We can thus say that there is a statistical difference in the diastolic blood pressure between the measurement time intervals.

Therefore we reject the **null hypothesis** that there is *no* difference between the diastolic blood pressure of patients measured at ten minutes and two hours after arrival at the out-patients' clinic. We conclude that a time interval of one hour and fifty minutes between an initial blood pressure measurement on arrival at the clinic and a subsequent measurement leads to a significantly different result being recorded.

Bigger or smaller: one or two tails?

One aspect of statistical testing that always tends to add confusion is the problem of tails. You may see written 'We use a two-tailed *t* test' but what does it mean? Let's recall the normal distribution from the study in Chapter 10. As with all normal-like distributions it has tails, two of them (see Figure 11.4). This is where the term 'two-tailed test' comes from. But what does it mean?

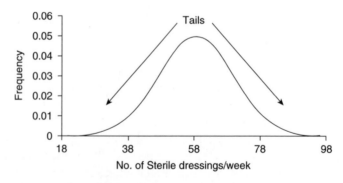

Figure 11.4   Distribution with two tails

Box 11.9

Recap.

- Use the z and t tests when you are looking to see if there is a significant difference between the means of two samples.
- Use them only where the samples are normally distributed (z) or you suspect that the parent population is normally distributed.
- Use them only for variables that are measured on the interval scale.
- Check that the variances are equal; use an F test for equality of variance.
- Decide whether or not you will opt for a one-tail or a two-tail test.

When we do a test we are trying to determine if our result is extreme and so are asking, does the test statistic or result lie in the tails of the distribution; does it fit? Does it belong with the distribution of this population or is it so extreme that in all probability it belongs with another?

Because the tails are at both ends it means we are looking for values both much smaller than the mean and much bigger. In which case, in terms of the hypotheses, we are simply looking for a difference, that is, the null hypothesis is that there is no difference. The alternative to the null, H_1, is that there is a difference.

But what if we suspect that our treatment (or intervention) will have a big effect in a particular direction, for example decrease the prevalence of a disease, increase the recovery rate. In many health care studies we are indeed looking for a difference in a particular direction. In the example above we are looking for extreme values in one end of the tail only. To convert from a two-tailed test to a one-tailed test is easy. Simply divide the probability level (P) by 2.

- If you are just looking for a difference use a two-tailed test.
- If you think your intervention will increase the measured variable, use a one-tailed test.
- If you think your intervention will decrease the measured variable, use a one-tailed test.

In the example used to explain the paired t test, clearly there is a prior belief that blood pressures recorded two hours after arrival will be lower than those recorded soon after arrival. This is a clear example where a one-tailed test could be used. When applied to the example the result is significant at a lower level of probability, that is, 0.01 divided by 2, which equals 0.005. Thus the result has a higher level of significance. In some cases the decision to use a one or two-tailed test can affect whether the null hypothesis is accepted or rejected. Therefore *if in doubt use a two-tailed test.*

Having read this chapter and completed the exercises, you should be familiar with the following ideas and concepts:

- How and when to perform an F test for equality of variance
- How and when to perform a z or student's t test
- How to perform a paired t test
- The rules that restrict the use of the t test
- The difference between a one and a two-tailed test
- When to use a one-tailed test
- When to use a two-tailed test

Exercises

1 Using the data from the second fictitious study (Symphadiol), plot a histogram using the descriptive statistics for weight loss for group 1 (control) and group 2.
2 State the hypothesis, and the null hypothesis.
3 You are looking to see if the weight loss of the treatment group is greater than that of the control: Perform an appropriate statistical test(s) on this sample.
4 Give your reasons for your choice of test.
5 State clearly the conclusions of your test.
6 Using the data below, suggest whether or not biology lectures had a significant impact on the performance of Year 1 Nursing Studies undergraduates in a biology examination. (a) What explanations could account for this result? (b) Do you think the lectures were of benefit? Should the students attend? (c) Did you use a one or two-tailed-test? Why?

	Exam Result	
Individual	before lectures	after lectures
1	34.5	37.5
2	37.2	40.2
3	43.0	42.0
4	48.8	51.8
5	49.6	52.6
6	50.8	50.8
7	51.2	54.2
8	51.5	54.5
9	52.5	55.5
10	63.4	62.4
11	64.6	67.6

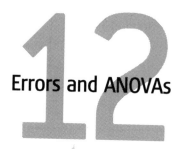

Errors and ANOVAs

Areas of learning covered in this chapter

What are	Type 1 and Type 2 errors?
What	can be done to reduce Type 1 errors?
How	are ANOVAs performed?
When do	I use a repeat measures design?

In the previous chapter we looked at tests based on the normal distribution designed to see if there is a difference between two treatment groups. But what if you have more than two groups? Say you have a control group and two different levels of a treatment. In that case you can't use a *t* test and must use a type of test that belongs to a group called **ANOVA**, which is shorthand for *analysis of variance*. There are several types of ANOVA but they have evolved to deal with a certain type of statistical error.

Statistical errors

If we choose the wrong type of statistical test we are likely to commit either a Type 1 or a Type 2 error. A **Type 1 error** occurs if you reject the null hypothesis when it should have been accepted. A **Type 2 error** is when a false null hypothesis is accepted. Type 1 and Type 2 errors are opposites. As you reduce the likelihood of a Type 1 the chance of a Type

2 increases. In general we tend to select tests that will *reduce* the chance of a Type 1, so a cautious approach is adopted. For example, we have said previously that in many medical studies the significance level is set at $P = 0.01$.

> Do not spend too much energy trying to remember which is which, just work on understanding what they mean. You can look up which is which when you need to.

Box 12.1

Errors

If you set your accepted value at 0.01 (1 per cent) you would have a 1 in 100 chance of getting it wrong. So an apparently simple solution is to increase the significance level. Unfortunately as Type 1 and Type 2 errors are opposites, as we decrease the chance of making a Type 1 error the chance of producing a Type 2 error increases.

---

t tests, errors and ANOVAs

We have said that you need an ANOVA when you have more than two groups. Let's look at why. Imagine we are doing a study where we have a control group (C) and two treatment groups (T1 and T2). We want to see if their means are significantly different; if we use a *t* test then we need to do several tests. We must test:

- C against T1.
- T1 against T2.
- T2 against C.

Perhaps this is not too much trouble if using a computer or even a calculator but if you had five treatment groups you would need to do ten tests. Even if you are prepared to stand the boredom, and manage not to make any calculation errors, you will commit a statistical error.

This is because: if you set your significance level at the normally accepted value of $P = 0.05$ (5 per cent), once every twenty tests (on average) you will get it wrong and commit a Type 1 error. But if, as in the case above, where we have five treatment groups, you perform ten *t* tests the chance of one of them being wrong goes up to one in two (that is, 0.05×10). So we need a way round this problem. The solution is to use an ANOVA.

ANOVA allows us to compare the means of several treatment groups at the same time without having to worry about adjusting *P* values or increasing the chance of Type 2 errors. It does this because it compares all the treatment groups in a single test. As you can imagine, the number of calculations needed to perform an ANOVA is quite large. However, with the advent of computers the use of ANOVA has become much more common and many more ANOVA-type tests have been designed. In this chapter we will look at two types of ANOVA.

Box 12.2

Robust and powerful

ANOVA is described as a *powerful* and *robust* technique. What do these terms mean?

The ANOVA

We will first describe the theory behind the ANOVA and then give one example, which we will work through. We will include the mathematical computation so that you can get an idea of how it works. In general it is better to use a computer, as they make fewer errors than humans. We suggest that you focus on the structure of the tests and interpreting the output. The type of ANOVA that we will describe is called the one-way analysis of variance.

Box 12.3

Computer statistics packages

SPSS, Minitab and Microsoft Excel can all help you to analyse data using the one-way ANOVA described here.

Criteria to be met before doing an ANOVA test

- The data of each treatment group are derived from a normal distribution.
- The data were measured on an interval/ratio scale.
- The variance between each group is not significantly different. (There are ways round this one.)
- The sample groups are measured **independently** of each other – see p. 126.

Box 12.4

What is meant by

- Normal distribution?
- Interval scale?
- Variance?

How does it work?

First, here are some data. The data set is smaller than would normally be used for ANOVA but we will use it to help us examine the ANOVA. The data in Table 12.1 are from a study to examine whether the pre-natal fitness level of Primip women significantly affects duration of labour. The term *Primip* denotes a woman who is in her first pregnancy. We want to compare the means of these three groups, but we can't use a *t* test. So we must opt for an ANOVA.

The ANOVA test looks at the source of variation in the overall data set and tries to apportion it to different aspects of the data. Once the variation has been allocated it is possible to see if the differences between the sample groups are significant. The sources of variation in the data are the variability that occurs *within* a sample group and the variability that occurs *between* the groups (Table 12.2).

> ANOVA seeks to determine how much of the variation in data sets can be attributed to error and how much can be attributed to the factor or treatment under study.

We can say that:

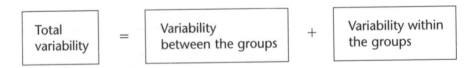

| Total variability | = | Variability between the groups | + | Variability within the groups |

We are interested in the between-group variation, that is, that which has occurred because of the fitness level. The rest of the variation, that is, that within the groups, we regard as error. The variability between groups will reflect the error that occurs within the groups and any additional variability caused by the treatment (in this case, fitness level).

Table 12.1   Duration of labour in Primip women aged between twenty-eight and thirty-two at three different levels of fitness

Fitness level 1	Fitness level 2	Fitness level 3
20	34	16
32	12	15
14	23	22
15	10	10

Level 1, low; level 2, medium; level 3, high.

Table 12.2   Variation within and between groups

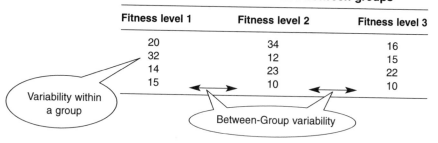

Fitness level 1	Fitness level 2	Fitness level 3
20	34	16
32	12	15
14	23	22
15	10	10

Variability within a group

Between-Group variability

If there is no difference between the groups, that is, the null hypothesis is correct, we would expect there to be just as much variation between the groups as there is within the groups. If the between-group variation is more than the within-group variation we know that the treatment has had an effect; and this is the simple logic behind the ANOVA test.

Box 12.5

- What are the causes of the within-group, variation, i.e. why do the cases of samples show variation?
- What are the causes of the between-group variation?
- What is F a measure of?

The test statistic produced by the ANOVA is F, a statistic we have seen before, and the measure of variation we use, the *variance*. Hence the name of the test: the analysis of variance.

If we compute the within-group variance and compare it with the between-group variance, F will equal 1 if the **null hypothesis** is correct. If F is significantly different from 1 we know that the means are significantly different, and the level of fitness (treatment groups) had an effect.

The procedure for calculating the ANOVA by hand is long-winded. It is probably worth doing by hand once or twice, as that will help you grasp how the procedure works and how ANOVAs are presented.

Table 12.3   Distance walked by patients (m) with impaired hip mobility, following various treatment regimes

Old frame		New frame	
	Exercise level 1	Exercise level 1	Exercise level 2
	16.1	22.3	13.2
	17.7	20.5	20.8
	20.6	21.3	22.2
	10.4	26.7	16.3
	20.3	16.3	13.7
	14.9	29.0	11.9
	11.5	24.4	14.1
	14.7	23.7	10.6
	15.3	23.5	15.8
	17.4	19.5	15.9
Mean	15.89	22.72	15.46
Standard deviation	3.32	3.63	3.67

Box 12.6

When to use a one-way ANOVA

When:

- You are comparing the difference between more than two sample groups.
- The data in each of your groups are normally distributed.
- Your data are measured on an interval scale.
- Each case is measured independently.

Example

In this example Martha Jones, a physiotherapist, is interested in the impact of the use of a new walking frame on her clients with impaired hip mobility. She has decided to test the new frame at two levels of exercise and use her old frame with the normal level of exercise as a control. Martha uses the distance the patient can walk unassisted as a measure of the effectiveness of the treatments (Table 12.3). Again, we will assume that the data are normally distributed, and remember that it would be normal to plot out the data to look for any odd results and get a 'feel' for your results.

Place the data into a table and, using a scientific calculator (if you have one), calculate the mean, the standard deviation, the variance, the sum of the cases and the sum of the cases squared (Table 12.4). Now we need to make sure that the variances of our sample groups are not significantly different, see criterion 3. To do this, select the largest and

Table 12.4   Statistical summary of the data from Table 12.3

	New frame		
Group 1 (GP1) Old frame	Group 2 (GP2) Exercise Level 1	Group 3 (GP3) Exercise Level 2	Total
12.1	22.3	13.2	
15.7	20.5	20.8	
18.6	21.3	22.2	
9.4	26.7	16.3	
18.3	16.3	13.7	
12.9	29.0	11.9	
9.5	24.4	14.1	
12.7	23.7	10.6	
13.3	23.5	15.8	
15.4	19.5	15.9	
$n = 10$	$n = 10$	$n = 10$	$n_{tot} = 30$
$\bar{x} = 13.79$	$\bar{x} = 22.72$	$\bar{x} = 15.46$	
$s = 3.21$	$s = 3.63$	$s = 3.67$	
$s^2 = 10.27$	$s^2 = 13.15$	$s^2 = 13.45$	
$\Sigma x = 137.9$	$\Sigma x = 227.2$	$\Sigma x = 154.6$	$\Sigma x_{tot} = 519.70$
$(\Sigma x)^2 = 19{,}016.4$	$(\Sigma x)^2 = 51{,}619.8$	$(\Sigma x)^2 = 23{,}890.8$	
$\Sigma x^2 = 1{,}994.11$	$\Sigma x^2 = 5{,}280.36$	$\Sigma x^2 = 2{,}762.4$	$\Sigma x^2_{tot} = 10{,}036.9$

smallest variances and perform an F test as in Chapter 10. There is no significant difference in the variances, so we can proceed with the test. The ANOVA test uses the sums of squares as a measure of variation, first seen in Chapter 6.

Step 1. Calculate a correction factor (CF). This makes the calculations a little quicker:

$$CF = \frac{\left(\sum x_{tot}\right)^2}{n_{tot}} = \frac{(519.70)^2}{30} = \frac{270{,}088.09}{30} = 9{,}002.93$$

Step 2. Calculate the sums of squares (SS) for the whole sample:

$$SS_{tot} = \sum x^2_{tot} - CF = 10{,}036.9 - 9{,}002.9 = 1{,}034$$

Step 3. Calculate the between groups sums of squares:

$$SS_{between} = \frac{\left(\Sigma x_{GP1}\right)^2}{n_{GP1}} + \frac{\left(\Sigma x_{GP2}\right)^2}{n_{GP2}} + \frac{\left(\Sigma x_{GP3}\right)^2}{n_{GP3}} - CF$$

$$SS_{between} = \frac{19{,}016.4}{10} + \frac{51{,}619.8}{10} + \frac{23{,}890.8}{10} - CF$$

$$SS_{between} = 1{,}901.6 + 5{,}161.9 + 2{,}389.1 - 9{,}002.93$$

$$SS_{between} = 449.67$$

Step 4. Calculate within-group sums of squares. A short cut can be used here because we know the between-group sums of squares and the total and we know that the between-groups and within-groups sums of squares must add up to the total:

$$SS_{total} = SS_{between} - SS_{within}$$

So:

$$SS_{within} = SS_{total} - SS_{between}$$
$$584.33 = 1,034 - 449.67$$

If you are forced to do ANOVAs by hand it's probably best to calculate both the within-group and the between-group sums of squares by long-hand. This will allow you to check your maths.

Step 5. Determine the degrees of freedom for both the within and between groups following the following rules.

$$\text{d.f. for } SS_{between} = \text{number of groups} - 1$$
$$(\text{In this example } 3 - 1 = 2)$$
$$\text{d.f. for } SS_{within} = \text{total number of cases} - \text{number of groups}$$
$$(\text{In this example } 30 - 3 = 27)$$
$$\text{d.f. for } SS_{total} = \text{d.f.}_{SSbetween} + \text{d.f.}_{SSwithin}$$

Step 6. Calculate the variances for both the between- and the within-group sums of squares:

$$S^2 \text{ between} = \frac{SS_{between}}{d.f._{between}} = \frac{449.67}{2} = 224.83$$

$$S^2 \text{ within} = \frac{SS_{within}}{d.f._{within}} = \frac{584.33}{27} = 21.64$$

Step 7. Calculate *F*:

$$F = \frac{\text{Variance between groups}}{\text{Variance between groups}} = \frac{224.83}{21.64} = 10.38$$

Step 8. It is normal for the results from an ANOVA to be put in a table laid out in a standard format like Table 12.5. The results of ANOVAs performed using statistical packages are often presented in such tables. An alternative would be Table 12.6.

Table 12.5

Source of variation	Sums of squares	d.f.	Variance	F
Between groups	449.67	2	224.83	10.38
Within groups	584.33	27	21.64	
Total	1,034	29		

Table 12.6

Source of variation	Sums of squares	d.f.	Mean squares	F
Between groups	449.67	2	224.83	10.38
Error	584.33	27	21.64	
Total	1,034	29		

Step 9. Look up the value of F in the appropriate statistical table (Appendix 2, Table 1). Note that the variance between groups should always be on top, and larger than the within-group variance. If the between-group variance is less than the within-group variance the null hypothesis is automatically accepted.

The value of 10.38 is significant at the $P < 0.01$ level and so we can reject the null hypothesis and say that the difference between the groups is significantly different. We would express this result by saying that there was a significant difference between the three treatment groups (ANOVA $F_{2, 27} = 10.38$, $n = 30$, $P < 0.01$.). Unlike the t test we also give the degrees of freedom for both within and between groups. They are given as a subscript to the F statistic.

Box 12.7

Performing an ANOVA

- Using the data from the Symphadiol study presented in Chapter 5, perform an ANOVA on the four treatments groups.
- Are the means significantly different?
- Did you look at plots of the data?
- What do you conclude?

Contrasting the means

You may have noted that there is a slight problem with the ANOVA in that, whilst we can say that there is a significant difference between the

Table 12.7   Comparing means after an ANOVA test

Group means	Group 1: 13.79	Group 2: 22.72	Group 3: 15.46
Group 1: 13.79		9.05	1.67
Group 2: 22.72			7.26
Group 3: 15.46			

sample groups, we can't say which groups are different from each other and which are not. Thus in the first example we do not know if both exercise regimes are both different from the control, or if they are different from each other, etc. Fortunately we can do follow-up tests that allow us to determine which sample groups are significantly different from each other.

For those using computer packages there are a range of these follow-up test options with an assortment of names. The only one to avoid is the least significant difference test, as you will make the same error as if you did multiple t tests. The most conservative (tends towards a Type 2 error) is Scheffe's test, the least conservative (tends towards a Type 1 error) is Duncan's multiple range test (Kerr, Hall and Kozub 2002). We will look at how one of these tests is calculated, namely the Tukey test. You need to do this test only if the result of your ANOVA test is significant.

Tukey test

Step 1. First compute a test statistic called T:

$$T = (q) \times \sqrt{\frac{\textit{Within-groups mean squares}}{n}}$$

You know the within-groups mean squares and can find it in your previous calculations. You can find q only by consulting a table showing the probability distribution of q. To find q you need to know the d.f. for the within-groups variance (called v in most statistical tables) and the number of sample groups (called k in most statistical tables). In our example:

$$T = (2.90) \times \sqrt{\frac{21.64}{10}} = 2.90 \times 1.47 = 4.26$$

Step 2. For each group mean compute the difference between it and each other group mean. You could use a table like Table 12.7.

Step 3. Compare the difference between each pair of means with the value of T. If the difference is larger, then the difference between the two means is statistically significant.

Box 12.8

Now, think about what you can conclude from this study:

- Which means are significantly different from each other?
- What do you conclude? Is the conclusion different now that you have contrasted the means?
- Would you make any recommendations based on the outcome of this study?

Independence

We said at the start of this chapter that for an ANOVA to be suitable the individual cases must be independent. What does that mean? Independence means that there should be no way the measurements from one individual measurement can interfere with or be affected by other measurements. For example, if you were issuing a questionnaire to two groups of people and it was possible that the two groups could talk to each other to discuss the questions, clearly the samples would not be independent. Of course, in some cases sample groups may contain the same individuals, particularly when you are following the response of individuals to a treatment. Here you must opt for a repeat measure design.

Box 12.9

- Using the results from the exercise in Box 12.7, perform a Tukey test.
- Which means are significantly different from each other?
- What do you conclude? Is the conclusion different now that you have contrasted the means?
- Would you make any recommendations based on the outcome of this study?

Repeat measure design of ANOVA

The repeat measure design should be used in any study where the same individual is tested more than once. It is analogous to the paired *t* test. Such tests are also known as within-group tests. We will look at the within-group one-way ANOVA. For this test we will simply look at the theory and at an ANOVA table. Worked examples can be found in texts such as Kerr *et al.* (2002).

If you design an experiment such that you follow a number of individuals, it stands to reason that you will have less variation caused by sampling

Table 12.8 Diastolic blood pressure of four men aged between fifty-six and fifty-eight at the start of and during a prescribed exercise regime

Individual	At start	After three weeks	After six weeks
1	92	89	85
2	94	87	84
3	90	92	90
4	97	96	92

Variability within a group

Reduced between-Group variability

error between the groups. Because you are using the same individuals in each sample group, the error between them is the same no matter which sampling group they are actually in. There will still be, of course, error due to intra-individual variation and random factors. (If there was no sampling error there would be much less need for statistics!)

> The sampling unit does not have to be a person, but the measurement must be made on the same object more than twice.

As you have less sampling error to deal with, you can use a smaller sample size. This is a major advantage of repeat measure experimental designs. If you just used a 'normal' ANOVA you would end up overestimating the between-group error and so would be more likely to produce a Type 2 error.

An example of a repeat measure design is shown in Table 12.8. It represents the diastolic blood pressure of four men who have been given a regime of exercise to follow as part of a treatment for mild hypertension. Each participant was measured at the start of the exercise programme and at three and six weeks after the start.

To take account of this reduced between-group error, the calculation of F is slightly altered so that the error due to difference in the individuals is not taken into account when we compare the groups. To do this, the within-group error is divided into two components. That due to the individuals is called the sums of squares of the subjects and the residual variation is the sums of squares. In other words:

$$SS_{Within\ Groups} = SS_{Subjects} + SS_{Residual}$$

If we can determine the $SS_{Subjects}$ then we can remove it, and the $SS_{Within\ Groups}$ used in the first ANOVA we described will be replaced by the term $SS_{Residual}$.

Fortunately we are able to compute $SS_{Subjects}$ and therefore perform a repeat measures ANOVA. However, we will not detail its calculation here.

Table 12.9

Source of variation	Sums of squares	d.f.	Mean squares	F
Between groups	61.17	2	30.58	5.58
Residual error	32.83	6	5.47	

When a repeat measure design is computed the ANOVA table will look like Table 12.9. This ANOVA has been generated for the data presented in table 12.8. Again you now must look to see if F is significant; P in this case is 0.043 (we used SPSS to calculate this). In other words $P < 0.05$, so the difference is significant.

If you have used a computer package you may well see reference to a phenomenon called **sphericity**. Sphericity, in the statistical sense, is the assumption that the variance of the differences between the experimental groups is not different. For most repeat measure design ANOVAs we must assume sphericity, and computer packages will perform a test of this assumption.

Having read this chapter and completed the exercises, you should be familiar with the following ideas and concepts:

- When to perform a one-way ANOVA
- When to use a repeat measures design one-way ANOVA
- How to perform a one-way ANOVA
- The rules that restrict the use of the ANOVA
- How to contrast the means following a one-way ANOVA

Exercises

1 Using the data from the study of Symphadiol in Chapter 5, plot a histogram using the descriptive statistics for group 1 (control), group 2, group 3 and group 4.
2 Plot a graph comparing these data, show the standard errors.
3 State the hypothesis of the experiment.
4 State the statistical and null hypotheses.
5 Perform an appropriate statistical test(s) (a) by hand, (b) using a computer package.
6 Compare the results. Which approach do you prefer and why?
7 What can you conclude about the impact of Symphadiol?
8 Collect a suitable data set of your own to perform an ANOVA. Remember the restrictions of this technique.

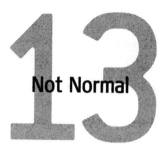

Not Normal

In the chapters on comparing differences you will have seen that most of the tests require your data set to be normally distributed, or at least not significantly different from normal (Chapter 10). This chapter addresses two problems: first, how do I know if my data are significantly different from normal and what do I do if they are?

If you look at the chapter on *t* tests (Chapter 11) you will see that sometimes because the data set is small you have to rely on an assumption that the data set will be normal, just because of the type of measurement it is. Measurements of human growth and development, for example, tend to be normally distributed. Similarly, other data such as percentages or counts of things you can probably say won't be normal. But what if you are unsure about what is 'normal'? What do you do then?

Of course, the first thing you should do is plot your data as a frequency histogram. If your data set is of thirty or more cases and your plot doesn't look normally distributed you can safely assume that it isn't. But what if, after doing your plot, you're still unsure? In that case you need to perform a statistical test, a test to tell you whether or not your data are significantly different from normal.

If you find that your data are *not* normally distributed you have two options: either transform the data, such that a parametric test is suitable, or use a **non-parametric** alternative (Chapter 14). You will want to use parametric tests if you can, because they are more robust and powerful than the non-parametric alternative. Parametric tests are based on probability distributions, non-parametric tests are not.

Box 13.1

What do the terms *skew* and *kurtosis* refer to?

If you are using a computer, there are several easily accessible tests available. We shall discuss the variety of options available to you. If you don't have a statistical package available, you will probably want to use a test called the χ^2 (chi square) test for goodness of fit. If, on the other hand, you do have access to a stats package then something like the Kolmogrov-Smirnov (KS) test, the Cochran test or tests for skewness and kurtosis will probably be more straightforward. Do not ignore the goodness of fit test, as it is useful, particularly when looking to see if data fit other distribution types.

Test for normality

Both the KS test and Cochran's compare the tested distribution against standards. These tests produce a test statistic and like any other if the test statistic exceeds the critical value then your distribution is significantly different from normal. Most computer packages will report the test statistic and calculate a P value. All you need to do is spot if the P value is less than $P = 0.05$. If it is, then your distribution is significantly different from normal.

Box 13.2

Test procedure for kurtosis and skewness

A test can be performed similar to the z test to determine if a distribution is significantly skewed or shows significant kurtosis. For any given frequency distribution a z score (termed z_{skew} or $z_{kurtosis}$) for both skewness and kurtosis can be calculated. If either of these values exceeds 1.96, the distribution in question can be said to differ significantly from normal. You then have two options, either transform your data to make them normal or use a non-parametric test (see Chapter 14).

Tests for skewness and kurtosis on the other hand look at your distribution to see if it is significantly more kurtosed or skewed, taking each of these measures one at a time.

Goodness of fit

The goodness of fit test that we will describe is based on the χ^2 distribution. Many statistics texts recommend using the G test instead of the χ^2 as it is more reliable. However, here we will stick to the χ^2 as few computer programmes support the G test and we discuss the χ^2 test elsewhere in this book. For a detailed discussion of the G test see Sokal and Rohlf (1996).

A goodness of fit test compares the distribution of numbers in a sample against a model distribution; if we are testing to see if your distribution is normal then the model distribution will be the normal distribution. The goodness of fit test can be used to test if your data fit any particular distribution. Thus they can be used to see if data fit other theoretical populations such as the Poisson or the binomial distributions.

> **A warning**
>
> If you are doing your statistics by hand, think twice about using a goodness of fit test to see if a normal distribution is appropriate. The process takes time and is tedious. Instead you could plot out your data and you could look to see if the data look normal. In addition you could estimate if 70 per cent of the cases lie within the bounds of the mean ± 1 SD.
>
> If your work is for publication it is likely, however, that some sort of test for normality will be required. An alternative would be to opt to use a non-parametric test that does not make assumptions about the distribution of the data.

For a goodness of fit test, we regard the sampled data as the 'observed data' and the model distribution as the 'expected'. We are testing to see if the observed frequency matches that predicted by the model distribution. For each observed case it is possible to predict how often it should occur theoretically and compare it with how often it actually does. The symbol f is used to denote frequency. Comparing observed results against expected results is the essence of the χ^2 test. For the normal distribution, the model equation that is used to predict the frequency for any given case (x) is shown below.

$$y = \frac{1}{\sigma\sqrt{(2\Pi)}} e^{-[(x-\mu)^2/2\sigma^2]}$$

In this equation there are two constants (values that don't change): e and π; the value of e is 2.71 and that of π, 3.1417. x stands for the value of a particular case, μ stands for the population mean and σ for the population standard deviation. Of course, because more often than not we are dealing with samples of populations, we have to use $\bar{x}$ and s as estimates of μ and σ. This gives rise to a slight problem in that we are trying to establish a model normal distribution, and in order to do that we need to be reasonably sure that our measures of $\bar{x}$ and s are reasonable estimates μ and σ. For this to be true, we need to have a *sample size more than thirty.*

The chi-square bit

We can predict 'expected' from our model distribution and as we have our own observed data we are in a position to perform a χ^2 (chi square) test (Chapter 15). The formula for a χ^2 is as follows:

$$\chi^2 = \sum \frac{(O - E)^2}{E}$$

The test statistic is χ, O stands for observed and E for expected. Σ of course stands for 'sum of'. What do we sum? We sum each occurrence where we can compare an observed with an expected result.

Example

Janet Thompson is doing a small research project looking at the number of visits made to a walk-in treatment centre by different sections of the community. She uses a period of a week as her sampling unit and wants to compare the frequency of visits of White European, Afro-Caribbean and Bangladeshi women. She suspects that as her data are counts of things her data samples may not be normally distributed. However, she wants to use parametric statistics, as she knows that these are more powerful and robust than the non-parametric alternatives.

She plots each of her cases. We will concentrate on the data for the Afro-Caribbean women. Are these data normally distributed? Looking at Figure 13.1, we can say that the graph does seem a little skewed; there are more points below the mean than above it. The mean of the data is 28.4 and the standard deviation is 13.90. The variance (standard deviation squared) is thus much larger than the mean and suggests that the data are positively skewed.

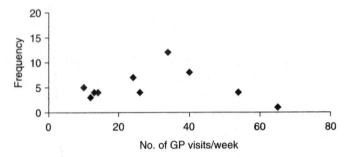

Figure 13.1   Frequency distribution of visits to a walk-in treatment centre by Afro-Caribbean women

Table 13.1   Calculating the standard deviation (S) and mean from a frequency table

No. of visits (x)	Frequency of visits(f)	Total no. of each class of visit (fx)	$(x - \bar{x})^2$	$f(x - \bar{x})^2$
34	12	408	31.7	381.0
12	3	36	267.8	803.5
65	1	65	1,342.1	1,342.1
13	4	52	236.1	944.4
10	5	50	337.3	1,686.4
54	4	216	657.1	2,628.5
24	7	168	19.1	133.4
40	8	320	135.3	1,082.9
26	4	104	5.6	22.4
14	4	56	206.4	825.5
	$n = 52$	$\Sigma fx = 1,475$	$\bar{x} = \Sigma fx/n = 28.4$	$\Sigma f(x - \bar{x})^2 = 9,850.1$
				$s = 13.90$

Box 13.3

Look back at Chapter 6 to see how to plot a frequency histogram.

When you have formulated your data into a frequency table, a quick method of calculating the mean can be seen in Table 13.1. The standard deviation can be calculated as:

$$s = \sqrt{\frac{\Sigma f(x - \bar{x})^2}{n - 1}}$$

Table 13.2   The observed and expected (as predicted by the normal distribution) frequency of visits to a walk-in treatment centre by Afro-Caribbean women

No. of visits	10	12	13	14	24	26	34	40	54	65
Actual frequency of that number of visits	5	3	4	4	7	4	12	8	4	1
Expected frequency	1	1	1	1	1.5	1.5	1.5	1	0.5	0.5

The sample mean is 28.4 and the standard deviation 13.9.

Now that you know the standard deviation the figures can be entered into the equation that will predict the frequency of any case for a given mean and standard deviation if the numbers are drawn from a normal distribution. For our data the actual frequencies are given in Table 13.2.

Box 13.4

Why are the expected values so low?

Note that you do not convert the actual values into percentages. To obtain the expected frequencies you must multiply the predicted frequency for each value of x by n. Notice how low the predicted values compare with the expected ones.

You are now in a position to do the actual goodness of fit test. For each value of x, perform the equation:

$$\frac{(O - E)^2}{E}$$

For the first value, this will be

$$\frac{(5 - 1)^2}{1}$$

which gives a value of 16. Repeat this for each value of x and then add together all the results. You should get:

$$16 + 4 + 9 + 9 + 20.2 + 4.2 + 73.5 + 49 + 24.5 + 0.5 = 209.9$$

i.e. $\chi^2 = 209.9$. As with most tests, you now have to look this value up in a table, using the appropriate degrees of freedom. The table is the χ^2

distribution table (Appendix 2). The degrees of freedom to use are the number of values − 2 (in this case 10 − 2). So we have eight degrees of freedom. The value in Table 4 for a level of significance of 0.05 is 15.51, therefore our value (being bigger than that in the table) indicates that the difference between the observed and the expected frequencies is significantly different and we can conclude that the distribution under investigation is significantly different from the normal distribution.

Box 13.5

Collect a sample of the shoe sizes of about thirty people. Determine if this sample is distributed in a manner that is significantly different from normal.

Using goodness of fit tests with the Poisson distribution

Goodness of fit can be used to see if frequency distributions fit any theoretical mathematical distribution of numbers. One important distribution for those working in health care is the Poisson distribution. It is a distribution that describes rare phenomena that occur in space or time randomly. For example, how many times does lightning strike per unit of time? We might want to ask whether or not the incidence of violent events in hospital A&E units is randomly dispersed across all hospitals in an area or are the events associated with something to do with that hospital? We might ask, does a disease such as myeloid leukaemia occur randomly across a particular country or is it associated with some other phenomenon such as the location? Because the Poisson distribution describes random distributions, we can use it to test if our data are randomly distributed or not. Test for a Poisson distribution if:

- Your data represent rare phenomena.
- The data consist of counts of things.
- The variance is quite similar to the mean.

The formula for predicting the probability of finding x number of occurrences of the rare phenomenon in a given sample is:

$$P_{(x)} = e^{-\bar{x}} \cdot \frac{\bar{x}^x}{x!}$$

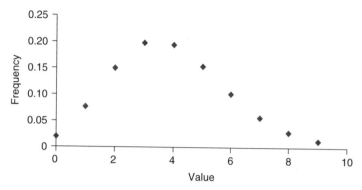

Figure 13.2   Poisson distribution

Who said life would be simple! By computer it is possible to extract these values more easily. Most of the mathematical functions in the equation you have seen before, with the exception of $x!$. The symbol ! means 'factorial'. The factorial of 3 would be the product of $1 \times 2 \times 3 = 6$. The factorial of 5 would be $1 \times 2 \times 3 \times 4 \times 5 = 120$. The · is shorthand for multiply, e is of course 2.71 (the base of the natural logarithm). So if $x = 3$ and the mean of your sample is 6:

$$P_{(3)} = e^{-\bar{6}} \cdot \frac{6^3}{3!} = 0.091$$

In other words, if the phenomenon is randomly distributed we have a 9.1 per cent chance of obtaining a value of 3.

We will use an example to demonstrate. Eastern Health Authority is concerned about recent outbreaks of MRSA in a number of wards. It is believed that there may be some link between outbreaks in different wards in different hospitals. The infection control officers sample forty wards across their area and record the number of patients who have apparently contracted an MRSA infection whilst in hospital. The frequencies of infection they find are shown in Table 13.3. The average number of infections per ward is 3.75. As with the example from the normal distribution, you now use a mathematical model, the Poisson distribution, to predict the expected frequency for this mean. As before, having found the expected frequency you can now perform a χ^2 test for goodness of fit.

In this case $\chi^2 = 9.22$. The degrees of freedom = the number of values -2, so in this case we have $10-2 = 8$. With eight degrees of freedom

Table 13.3   The observed and expected (as predicted by the Poisson distribution) of the number of MRSA infected patients across wards

No. of infected patients	0	1	2	3	4	5	6	7	8	9
Frequency	3	3	5	6	6	5	3	2	2	1
Expected frequency	0.7	3.0	6.0	7.9	7.8	6.2	4.1	2.3	1.1	0.5

the critical value in the χ^2 distribution table is 15.51 at $P = 0.05$. As our calculated value of χ^2 is less than 15.51 we can say that there is no significant difference between the observed values and those predicted by the Poisson distribution. We can therefore conclude that the occurrences of MSRA in the Eastern Health Authority show a distribution that is not significantly different from random.

Transforming

If you have tested your data and they are not normal, the rest of this chapter devotes itself to what to do next.

What is a transformation?

Simply put, a transformation is where we alter the distribution of a set of data by applying a mathematical function to each case. We might, for example, square-root each case. If this sounds like fiddling your data, it isn't: transformations have been used for years and their soundness has been tested over time. For most of the common deviations from the normal distribution there is a standard transformation. Here we will describe three types of transformation: the logarithmic, the arcsine and the square root. These are probably the most common.

The logarithmic transformation

We use a logarithmic (log.) transformation where it is noticed that the variance of the samples increases with the mean, where the data are clumped (there is a large frequency of cases against just one or two values) or where the frequency distribution is skewed to the right.

> ## Box 13.6
>
> When should you quote a standard error?

To perform a log transformation, simply log all the cases. You then per-form the appropriate statistical test on the logged data. Having logged the data, you should, of course, check that the new distribution isn't significantly different from normal. Do not forget that the standard error and confidence limits rely on the data set being normal. If you want to quote these values you must first calculate the values using the transformed data, and then antilog the values to obtain quotable mean-ingful figures. With all transformations, you must reverse the transfor-mation in order to report means, standard errors and confidence limits.

If your data are composed of counts of something and you have a lot of zeros, try using log $(x + 1)$, that is, add one to each case and then log the result.

The arcsine transformation

This transformation is useful for data that have been recorded as percent-ages or proportions. It is sometimes called the angular transformation. The formula for the arcsine transformation is:

$$TV = \arcsin \sqrt{p}$$

where TV stands for the transformed value and p for a proportion.

If the cases of your data have been measured as a proportion (a percentage is simply a special type of proportion: divide by 100 and then proceed) then every case represents a p. If the cases in your sample fall in the range of 0.30 – 0.70 (30 per cent to 70 per cent) there is nor-mally no need to transform the data.

In order to perform an arcsine transformation first square-root all your samples, then obtain the angle of the sine of the resultant. On a calculator, use the inverse sine (sin[1] key). The answer should be expressed in degrees.

To convert back to normal values, again take each transformed value, find its sine and square this value (Fowler and Cohen 1990).

The square root transformation

If your samples are Poisson-distributed (the variance is similar to the mean) you will need to use the square root transformation. As the name of this transformation suggests, each case should be square-rooted, then the statistical test applied. Values can be squared to report the mean, standard error and confidence limits. If the data contain zeroes, rather than take the square root take the square root of (x + 0.5), that is, add 0.5 to each case then square-root it.

For a thorough discussion of transformations see Sokal and Rohlf (1996).

Having read this chapter and completed the exercises, you should be familiar with the following ideas and concepts:

- Why transformations are used
- How to use a χ^2 test for goodness of fit
- Poisson distribution
- The logarithmic, arcsine and square root transformations

Exercises

1   Using the data on age from the questionnaire (Chapter 5), perform an appropriate test to see if these data are normally distributed. Note: this is difficult without the help of a statistical package.
2   What type of distribution does the variable 'number of partners' have? Can you transform these data to make them follow a normal distribution? Why might you want to?

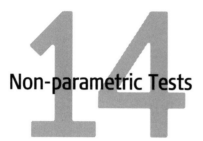

Non-parametric Tests

Areas of learning covered in this chapter

What are   non-parametric tests?
When should   non-parametric tests be used ?
What types of basic non-parametric test are there?

Up to now we have described tests that are known as *parametric* tests. These tests rely on the data being distributed in a certain way (quite often, normally). Parametric tests are thought to be the most powerful tests, as they allow very in-depth statistical interrogation and testing of data. Unfortunately a substantial number of the data we collect in relation to health care research are not normally distributed and our ability to transform such data to a normal distribution is limited (see Chapter 13). This chapter will introduce a range of tests that do not rely on the data conforming to a certain distribution. As such they can be used with data that are not normally distributed. They are known as non-parametric tests. We have already come across one group of non-parametric tests, those that use the χ^2 statistic. This chapter will describe some of the non-parametric tests that are analogous to the parametric tests described in this book.

Health care research often involves us working as social scientists. We are often involved in collecting a wide range of quantitative data. We are often interested in variables that are measured on the ordinal scale (for example, perceived amount of pain, anxiety state) or the nominal scale

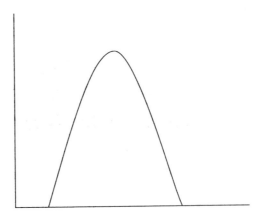

Figure 14.1   Normal distribution

(for example, profession, type of education, housing type, ethnic group).
Such variables are less likely to be normally distributed and therefore
you will need to be familiar with non-parametric tests.

When to use non-parametric tests

Non-parametric tests should be used when the data do not conform to
the conditions required for a parametric test. Normally, when we consider population distributions, we use such parameters as the mean or
the standard deviation. This is fine if the distribution of your data is
normal. However, in distributions that are not normally distributed
(Figure 14.1) but skewed (Figure 14.2) or distributed in some other way
(see Chapter 13), and the mean is not an appropriate descriptive test to use
(see Chapter 6), then a nonparametric test is probably more appropriate.

Non-parametric tests can also be used on small samples; we have
described a parametric test, the student's t test, that is appropriate for
small samples. If, however, you are unsure that the data collected will
conform to a normal distribution and your sample is small then it is
safer to opt for a non-parametric test.

Non-parametric tests are normally used for data collected using the
ordinal and nominal scales of measurement. However, they can also be
used for interval and ratio measurements where the distribution does
not conform to normality.

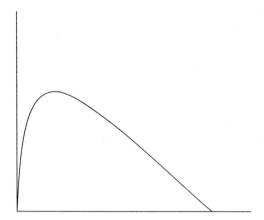

Figure 14.2   Skewed distribution

Non-parametric tests are not based on distributions, but on exact probabilities. They do not use the mean, but are more likely to be based on comparing the extent to which data deviate from the median. As such, when using non-parametric tests it is more appropriate to quote the median.

Box 14.1

Choice of Statistic

Review three or four research articles that use a statistical approach:

- See if you can spot the type of statistic used (parametric or non-parametric).
- Discuss the justification used for that particular choice.

Finally, non-parametric tests can be conducted on data from subjects that have not been randomly selected from the population from which they derive. In health care research it can be difficult to achieve a random sample because samples are often convenience-based and as such not randomly drawn from the population. Care must be taken, however, to bear this in mind when interpreting the results.

Box 14.2

Difference between Parametric and Non-parametric tests

Non-parametric	Parametric
• Can be used on ordinal and nominal scale data (although also on interval and ratio scale).	• Used mainly on interval and ratio scale data.
• Can be used on small samples.	• Tend to need larger samples.
• Can be used on data that are not normally distributed.	• Data should fit a particular distribution; the data can be transformed to that distribution.
• Can be used where the samples are not selected randomly.	• Samples should be drawn randomly from the population.
• Have less power than the equivalent parametric test.	• More powerful than non-parametric equivalent.

The principle behind using a non-parametric procedure as a statistical test is the same as for parametric procedures. You form a null hypothesis, gather your data, subject the data to the appropriate statistical equations (depending on the test chosen), produce a test statistic and, finally, see if your result is statistically significant by looking the result up in statistical tables using the appropriate degrees of freedom. Remember, we perform statistical tests so that we know that if we find a difference or a relationship we state that it is unlikely to have arisen by chance.

Ranking data

Many non-parametric tests involve ranking the data. In this section we explore this process. Ranking is simply a way of placing all the cases in order. For example, two groups of students watched a health promotion video and valued it out of 10, with 1 meaning 'poor' and 10 meaning 'excellent'. The students from school A gave the video values of 3, 5, 6 and 6. The pupils from school B gave it 1, 3, 6, 8. To rank these scores, first place all the numbers together in numerical order: 1, 3, 3, 5, 6, 6, 6, 8. We assign each a number that corresponds to its position in the original numerical line-up (order). We can then assign a rank to each score. If in

Table 14.1   Values that school children gave to a health promotion video

Value	1	3	3	5	6	6	6	8
Order	1	2	3	4	5	6	7	8
Rank	1	2.5	2.5	4	6	6	6	8

The values have been ordered and then ranked.

your data sets all the scores (values) occur only once then the rank will correspond to the order. Unfortunately in Table 14.1, as is common in most studies, some of our values occur more than once and as such we need to take this into account when determining the rank.

Box 14.3

Practise ranking

Ask 12 friends or colleagues to score on a scale of 1–10 the quality of the last meal that they bought. Ask another group to score on the same scale the last meal they made for themselves.

Order and rank each set of values.

Determining rank score

To do this, where a score (value) occurs more than once we add the order of those values together and divide by the number of times that the particular score (value) occurs. The result becomes the rank for that score (value). In Table 14.1 the value 3 occurs twice. The value 3 occupies two positions in the order, namely 2 and 3. To calculate rank we thus add 2 and 3 together, and divide by the number of times the value 3 occurs (2). Thus, the rank for the value 3 is 2.5. Repeating this for the other value where there is another tie (for the value 6), you get the ranks as shown in Table 14.1

The tests

Test for difference in two independent or unrelated samples: a substitute for the student's *t* test and the *z* test

The Mann–Whitney *U* test is a non-parametric test for differences in the **median** of two independent samples. As with the *t* test, 'independent'

Table 14.2   The attitude scores of people to the siting of an asylum centre in the vicinity of their village

West	East
1	2
2	3
2	3
3	5
5	6
5	8
6	8
6	9
7	9
7	10
7	
8	

score: 1 (very positive) to 10 (very negative).

means that the groups are not connected. You must have a set of data with regard to a parameter from one group of participants or objects and a second set from a different group.

The Mann–Whitney U test calculates the test statistic U. This statistic is then looked up in the appropriate statistical table and its significance determined. As with most statistical tests we start with a hypothesis. In Table 14.2, Marion Smith, a social worker, has measured the attitude of members of the public to having a reception centre for asylum seekers located in the vicinity of their village. She has scored attitudes on a 1–10 scale, with 1 being very positive and 10 very negative. She hypothesised before undertaking her study that people from West village would have a more negative attitude as that village is more affluent and people would be more concerned about the impact of the centre on property prices. Marion Smith is concerned the centre is located on a site that is sensitive to the views of the community, as this will influence the social well-being of both the asylum seekers and the villagers. The results of her study are shown in the table. The formula of the Mann-Whitney U test is as follows:

$$U_1 = n_1 \times n_2 + \frac{n_2(n_2+1)}{2} - R_2$$

$$U_2 = n_1 \times n_2 + \frac{n_1(n_1+1)}{2} - R_1$$

You can no doubt see that two values of U are calculated, U_1 and U_2. You will see later how these two values are used. $n1$ stands for the sample size of the first sample and n_2 for that of the second; R_1 is the sum of the ranks from the first sample and R_2 the sum of the ranks from the

> Remember that, to rank the data, both sets have to be arranged together. Do not rank groups separately.

second.

Table 14.3

Village	W	W	W	E	W	E	E	W	W	E	W	W	E	W	W	W	W	E	E	E	E	E
Value	1	2	2	2	3	3	3	5	5	5	6	6	6	7	7	7	8	8	8	9	9	10
Order	1	2	3	4	5	6	7	8	9	10	11	12	13	14	15	16	17	18	19	20	21	22
Rank	1	3	3	3	6	6	6	9	9	9	12	12	12	15	15	15	18	18	18	21.5	21.5	22

Step 1. Rank the data (Table 14.3). Note we have included an indication as to which village each value and rank came from. Also note that several of the values are repeated.

Table 14.4

Village	W	W	W		W			W	W		W	W		W	W	W	W					
Rank	1	3	3		6			9	9		12	12		15	15	15	18					

Village				E		E	E			E			E					E	E	E	E	E
Rank				3		6	6			9			12					18	18	21.5	21.5	22

Step 2. Separate out the ranks of each sample (Table 14.4).
Step 3. Sum the ranks for each sample (village). Sum of ranks for West village (ΣR_1): $1+3+3+6+9+9+12+12+15+15+15+18 = 118$. Sum of ranks for East village (ΣR_2): 137.

Box 14.4

A new descriptive statistic?

The sum of the ranks provides us with a descriptive of how different the two villages' attitudes to the asylum centre are. We can see that the sum of the ranks is 118 for West village and for East village it is 137. This indicates that West village has lower scores. If the two populations did not differ very much you would expect the scores to be similar and therefore not to be significantly different. The sum of ranks can be a useful descriptive statistic to present, as it provides a greater level of precision than the median.

Step 4. Load the values into the first equation:

$$U_1 = 12 \times 10 + \frac{10(10+1)}{2} - 137$$

$$U_1 = 120 + \frac{110}{2} - 137$$

$$U_1 = 120 + 55 - 137$$

$$U_1 = 38$$

Step 5. Repeat for the second equation:

$$U_2 = n_1 \times n_2 + \frac{n_1(n_1+1)}{2} - R_1$$

$$U_2 = 12 \times 10 + \frac{12(12+1)}{2} - 118$$

$$U_2 = 120 + 78 - 118$$

$$U_2 = 80$$

So $U_1 = 38$ and $U_2 = 80$. In the Mann-Whitney U test we are interested in the smallest value only, therefore for the purposes of this test $U = 38$.

Box 14.5

Finding the difference

For the data you obtained for the exercise in Box 14.3 perform a Mann–Whitney U test to see if there is a difference in the medians of the values.

What difficulties can you see in using scores of this nature?

We now must look this value up in the table of Mann-Whitney U values (Appendix 2, Table 6), using the sample sizes of 10 and 12 (as these were the sample sizes from the two villages). The critical value from the table is 29. As our value is greater than this, we are unable to reject the null hypothesis. *Note that this is the only test we have described so far in this book where if the critical value is exceeded the null hypothesis is not rejected.* Marion Smith concludes that there is no difference in the attitudes of the two villages towards the asylum centre.

You will notice that the Mann-Whitney U table does not exceed 20. At sample sizes above twenty the distribution of U begins to approximate to the normal distribution, and what this means in lay terms is that the normal distribution should be used instead (Fowler and Cohen 1990). To do this you must convert your U statistic to a t statistic, using the following formula:

$$t = \frac{U - (n_1 \times n_2)/2}{\frac{n_1 \times n_2 (n_1 + n_2 + 1)}{12}}$$

The calculated value of t can then be looked up in the t distribution tables.

Tests for differences between two related samples: the Wilcoxon two-sample test: a substitute for the paired T test

In the above example our two sets of data were not related, they were collected from two independent groups of students. There are many ways that data can be classified as related. For example, each person may be asked to evaluate two different forms of birth control. Consequently each person provides two pieces of data that are considered related. Equally, people may be paired by similar characteristics or sets of parameters. Finally there are before-and-after tests where once again one individual provides two pieces of data. In

Restrictions on the use of the Mann-Whitney U test

- Can be used on interval and ratio and ordinal scale data, as well as on proportions, percentages and counts.
- Samples or groups should come from data that have similar distributions, although they do not need to be the same.
- If your ranked data contain a large number of ties, a correction needs to be made. This correction is given automatically on most statistical packages.
- Can be used only to contrast two groups.

Table 14.5   Patient scores of quality of service before and after the practice nurse attended a training course

Patient	Before	After	Difference
1	2	8	−6
2	5	3	+2
3	6	5	+1
4	5	6	−1
5	9	4	+5
6	7	3	+4
7	8	1	+7
8	7	5	+2
9	6	3	+3
10	5	2	+3

Table 14.6   The differences in the scores of the pairs from Table 14.5, ordered and ranked

Difference	+1	−1	+2	+2	+3	+3	+4	+5	−6	+7
Order	1	2	3	4	5	6	7	8	9	10
rank	1.5	1.5	3.5	3.5	5.5	5.5	7	8	9	10

these cases it is not possible to use the Mann–Whitney U test but instead the Wilcoxon test can be used. The test statistic calculated in Wilcoxon's test is called T.

In Table 14.5 the manager of a general practice is evaluating the impact of an advanced practitioner training course on the perception of a group of patients of the quality of service given by the practice nurse. The manager decides to give a questionnaire to a group of ten patients who need to visit the nurse on a regular basis. He asks the patients to complete the questionnaire before and after the nurse has attended the course. As the same patients are used, the samples are related. As the measurement, in this case an evaluation of overall quality, was on the ordinal scale the manager selected the Wilcoxon two-sample test.

Once the data have been entered into a table (see Table 14.5), subtract one column from the other. It does not matter which set of data you enter in which column. The first step is to calculate the differences between each of the pairs, in this case the result before and the result after the training. The second is to rank the differences using the same techniques in the Mann-Whitney U test. When doing this, ignore any values where the difference is 0, and also use the absolute value of the difference, that is, ignore the signs at this stage (Table 14.6).

Step 3 is to sum the ranks where the difference has a negative sign, and then sum the ranks where the sum has a positive sign. Sum of the negative difference ranks: 1.5+9 = 10.5. Sum of the positive difference ranks: 1.5+3.5+3.5+5.5+5.5+7+8+10 = 44.5 Whichever sum is the smaller is given the value *T*. Therefore, in this case *T* = 10.5.

Having found the test statistic we now need to establish a value that is equivalent to the degrees of freedom in other tests. This value is called *N*. To calculate the value of *N* count the number of pairs of scores but subtract any whose difference is 0. In this case there were no differences of 0, therefore N = 10.

Box 14.6

One or two-tailed test.

Using your judgement decide if this test should be a one-tailed or a two-tailed test. Discuss the reasons why you have reached this conclusion.

Using the table of critical values of *T* (Appendix 2, Table 7) by locating the row where *N* = 10, the critical value is 10. In the Wilcoxon two-sample test, if the test statistic is equal or smaller (as with the Mann-Witney *U* test, this is the *opposite* of most statistical tests) than the critical value the result *is* significant. In this case 10.5 is not significant at the *P* < 0.05 level whether it is a one-tailed test or a two-tailed test.

Restrictions on the use of Wilcoxon's two-sample test

The Wilcoxon test makes the assumption that the samples have been drawn from populations that have a distribution that is symmetrical. In particular it should not be used where the distributions are skewed.

Test for difference in more than two independent or unrelated samples: a substitute for the one-way analysis of variance.

The Kruskal-Wallis *H* test is a test of significance used when there are more than two independent samples and when alternative parametric tests cannot be used. It can be used with data measured on the ordinal, interval or ratio scale.

In a previous example we compared the data from two villages with regard to their attitude to the siting of an asylum centre, but what if we

Table 14.7   The attitude scores of people to the siting of an asylum centre in the vicinity of their village

West	East	North
1	2	8
2	3	9
2	3	10
3	5	9
5	6	8
5	8	7
6	8	6
6	9	9
7	9	8
7	10	9
7		10
8		

Score: 1 (very positive) to 10 (very negative).

wanted to introduce a third sample, North village? We could conduct three Mann–Whitney *U* tests as outlined below:

School A by B.
School A by C.
School B by C.

The problem with this, however, is that there is an increased likelihood of producing a Type 1 error (just the same situation as if we were to perform multiple *t* tests, see Chapter 12). A Type 1 error is where the null hypothesis is rejected when it should have been accepted. The Kruskal-Wallis test is the non-parametric version. It should be used where you have two or more groups of data that are not normally distributed.

The Kruskal–Wallis test is very similar to the Wilcoxon test and also uses ranks. The test aims to determine if there are significant differences between the groups. It actually tests for a significant difference between the average rank.

In Table 14.7, Marion Smith has introduced a new village (North Village) into her sample, to analyse the data she needs to use a Kruskal-Wallis test.

As with the Wilcoxon test, the first step is to order and then rank the data (noting from which sample each of the ranks came from). See Table 14.8.

> Remember to combine all the groups when ranking the data; do not rank each group separately.

Table 14.8 The scores and ranks of the data presented in Table 14.7

West village		East village		North village	
Score	Rank	Score	Rank	Score	Rank
1	1	2	3	8	21.5
2	3	3	6	9	27.5
2	3	3	6	10	32
3	6	5	9	9	27.5
5	9	6	12.5	8	21.5
5	9	8	21.5	7	16.5
6	12.5	8	21.5	6	12.5
6	12.5	9	27.5	9	27.5
7	16.5	9	27.5	8	21.5
7	16.5	10	32	9	27.5
7	16.5			10	32
8	21.5				

Table 14.9 Statistical summary of the ranking data presented in table 14.8

	West	East	North
Sample size (n)	12	10	11
Sum of ranks (ΣR)	127	166.5	295
ΣR^2	16,129	27,722	87,025
$\Sigma R^2/n$	1,344	2,772	7,911

Having calculated the ranks, the next step is to calculate, for each sample (village) the sum of the ranks, the square of the sum of the ranks and $\Sigma R^2/n$. See Table 14.9.

Two more values that we need to know are N, which is the sum of the sample size (Σn), and also $\Sigma (\Sigma R^2/n)$ which is the sum of all the values in the final row of Table 14.9. In this case $N = 33$ and $\Sigma (\Sigma R^2/n) = 12,027$

The next step is to plug your values into the equation that produces the test statistic that in this case is called H:

$$H = \left[\Sigma(R^2/n) \times \frac{12}{N(N+1)} \right] - 3(N+1)$$

$$H = \left[12,027 \times \frac{12}{33 \times 32} \right] - 102$$

$$H = [12,027 \times 0.011] - 102$$

$$H = 30.29$$

Box 14.7

Kruskal-Wallis test

To the data you analysed in Box 14.5, ask another ten people to score the quality of the last meal they ate. Use a Kruskal-Wallis test to determine if the difference in the three groups is significant.

What potential problems can you see with this study?

Having found the test statistic H, we now must look this up in the appropriate table. In this case it is the distribution of χ^2. As this test uses the χ^2 distribution to find the appropriate critical value, we must first calculate the degrees of freedom used. They are calculated by taking the number of samples (in this case 3, i.e. three villages) and subtracting 1. Therefore in this example there are two degrees of freedom. At $P = 0.05$ the critical value is 5.99, the calcu-

Restrictions on the use of the Kruskal-Wallis test

If you are testing for differences between just three groups, you need to have data from at least five participants or objects for each group.

The data can be interval and ratio and ordinal-scale data, as well as proportions, percentages and counts.

lated value is *bigger* than this value, so in this case we reject the null hypothesis. *Note this is the same (that is, if the calculated value is bigger than the critical reject the null) as most other statistical tests but is the opposite of the two tests we have described in this chapter.* In theory a correction should be made in the calculation of H where there are ties. However, in practice this makes very little difference to the overall result.

Correlation: a substitute test for Pearson's correlation coefficient, the Spearman rank correlation

The Spearman rank correlation is a test that is used to determine the extent to which a change in one variable tends to be associated with a change in another. The correlation techniques we will look at test for linear correlation, that is, are the variables associated along a straight-line continuum? Where one variable is associated with another in this way they are said to be *correlated*. The Spearman rank can be used with data collected on ordinal, ratio and interval scales. It is ideal for use where sample sizes are small (less than twenty).

Table 14.10   The relationship between alcohol handrub use and incidence of MRSA in a Swiss hospital

Year	Alcohol-based handrub l/1000 patient days	New MRSA/100 admissions
1993	3.5	0.50
1994	4.1	0.60
1995	6.9	0.48
1996	9.5	0.32
1997	10.9	0.25
1998	15.4	0.26

When we perform a correlation, we not only ask if there is a correlation but we also want to know how strong the relationship is. The correlation test asks, how strong is the relationship and is the correlation greater than could be expected by chance? To perform a correlation you must have measures of two different variables from the same participant or object (see also Chapter 16).

In Table 14.10, we have taken data from Pittet *et al.* (2000), who investigated the effectiveness of a hospital-wide programme to improve compliance with hand hygiene. The aspect of this that we will look at is the relationship between the amount of alcohol handrub used per patient day and the incidence of hospital-acquired MRSA. The study was based on a Swiss hospital.

The research question is thus 'Is there a relationship between the amount of handrub used and the incidence of hospital acquired MRSA?', the hypothesis being that as more handrub is used the incidence of MRSA should decrease. There are insufficient data here to perform a Pearson correlation (Chapter 16). In addition, it is unlikely that the measurement of MRSA per patient would come from a normal distribution. Thus, a Spearman rank correlation is appropriate for these data.

The Spearman rank correlation

As the name implies, the Spearman rank correlation involves ranking the data. In the case of the Spearman rank correlation, each variable is ranked separately, and the difference between the rank for each pair of variables for each participant or 'object' is recorded. In Table 14.11 the 'object' is a year. As well as ranking the data we also need to calculate d^2 and Σd^2. In this case $\Sigma d^2 = 66$.

As normal, having done the basic calculation, now plug the values into the appropriate equation to produce the test statistic, in this case the Spearman rank correlation coefficient or r_s. The equation is:

Table 14.11 The data from table 14.10, showing ranks and differences between the ranks

Year	Alcohol-based handrub 1/1000 patient days	Rank	New MRSA/100 admissions	Rank	Difference in ranks (d)	d^2
1993	3.5	1	0.50	5	4	16
1994	4.1	2	0.60	6	4	16
1995	6.9	3	0.48	4	1	1
1996	9.5	4	0.32	3	1	1
1997	10.9	5	0.25	1	4	16
1998	15.4	6	0.26	2	4	16

$$r_s = 1 - \frac{6 \times \Sigma d^2}{n^3 - n}$$

In this case n is 6, as we have six samples.

$$r_s = 1 - \frac{6 \times 66}{(6 \times 6 \times 6) - 6}$$

$$r_s = 1 - \frac{396}{210}$$

$$r_s = -0.88$$

In correlation a value of 1 indicates a perfect positive relationship, whilst a value of −1 indicates a perfect negative relationship. A value of 0 would indicate that there was no relationship. Our value of −0.88 indicates that the two variables are negatively correlated, meaning that as one variable increases (the amount of handrub used) the other decreases (the MRSA infection rate). But is this correlation statistically significant? As normal, we turn to the appropriate statistical table (Appendix 2, Table 5). With a sample size of six, the critical value is 0.829 for a one-tailed test at

---

Restrictions on the use of the Spearman rank correlation

- As with all correlation techniques, a strong correlation does not mean that there is cause and effect.
- Once the sample size exceeds thirty, the result obtained using either the Pearson correlation or the Spearman rank correlation will be similar.
- If too many ranks are tied, error may be introduced into the calculation of r_s.

$P < 0.05$. Thus there is a statistically significant negative relationship between the amount of alcohol handrub used and the incidence of hospital-acquired MRSA.

Summary of tests

Table 14.12   Summary of tests

Name of test	Test is for	No. of samples/groups	Substitute for
Mann–Whitney U	difference in the medians of two unrelated/independent samples	2	t-test
Wilcoxon	difference in the medians of two related samples/paired samples	2	paired test
Kruskal–Wallis	difference in the medians of more than two unrelated/independent samples	3 or more	one way ANOVA
Spearman rank	correlations between two variables recorded from the same sampling unit.	1	person's correlation

All these tests can be used for variables where the measurement is recorded on the ordinal, interval or ratio scales.

Having read this chapter and completed the exercises, you should be familiar with the following ideas and concepts:

- The difference between parametric and non-parametric tests
- The types of data that can be investigated using basic non-parametric tests
- The type of statistical question that can be asked using basic non-parametric tests
- The Mann–Whitney U test
- The Wilcoxon test
- The Kruskal–Wallis test
- The Spearman rank correlation

Exercises

1 Using the data from the walk-in centre questionnaire, perform an appropriate test to see if there is a difference between the number of sexual partners of individuals from the Asian and African ethnic groups. What explanations do you think there are for the relationship?
2 Repeat question 1 above, only this time include the individuals from the European ethnic group.
3 Is there a significant decrease in the number of sexual partners with age?

Tests for Association (1) Chi-square

Areas of learning covered in this chapter

What are: tests for association and chi-square tests?
How are: chi-square tests used?
What types of: restrictions are there on the use of chi-square tests.

Tests for association

Sometimes when conducting studies we are interested in whether there is an association between two variables rather than a difference. For example, you may be interested to know if certain pathologies are associated with certain ethnic groups. Knowing such information would help with the planning of health care services and the development of public health campaigns. An example of such association is that between Afro-Caribbean communities and sickle-cell anaemia as is the association between cystic fibrosis and white Caucasian groups. When the association you are looking for involves data measured using the nominal scale it is normal to use chi-square tests.

    Other types of association are where we find that a change in one variable tends to be associated with a change in another. For example, there is an association between age and the occurrence of breast cancer. Sometimes we may find a decrease in one variable as another variable increases. For example, there is an association between increasing wealth and decreasing incidence of mental health problems. These types of association are known as *correlations*. Correlations normally involve using data that have been measured on the ordinal, interval or ratio scales. In this chapter we will look at the chi-square test and in Chapter 16 at correlations.

Box 15.1

When to use x^2

Use a x^2 test when:

- Your variables have been collected using a nominal scale.
- You want to see if there is an association between a variable and a particular phenomenon.

Do not convert your data to percentages prior to using the x^2 test.

The Greek letter chi is written x, thus the shorthand for chi-square is x^2. There are several forms of the x^2 test. They are, however, all based on the x^2 distribution and (although we use them to test for associations) are based on looking for a difference between what we expect to be the result and what we have actually observed. Chi-square tests are among the most widely used statistical tests. Chi-square tests always use data based on counts of either people or things. In this chapter we will look at two types of x^2 test: the one-way x^2 test and the x^2 test for association.

Chi-square test: one-way

This is probably one of the simplest statistical tests to perform and the basic calculation is:

$$x^2 = \sum \frac{(O - E)^2}{E}$$

The O stands for observed frequency and the E for the expected frequency. The Σ symbol means 'the sum of'. So x^2 is the sum of all the $(O - E)^2/E$ calculations. The important thing to remember about x^2 tests is that they use **frequencies** and if your data are not recorded or can't be converted into frequencies you can't use x^2 tests. The test is called a

Table 15.1   The ethnicity of individuals in a cohort entering nurse education

	White (UK and EU)	Caribbean	Indian subcontinent	Total (from these groups)
Observed	34	62	28	124

one-way test because there is just one variable involved (although this variable may be divided into several categories).

Box 15.2

Eye colour and chi-square tests

- Sample the eye colour of a group of individuals. Test to see if there is a significant association between eye colour and your sample group. Use a chi-square test for homogeneity.
- Is a chi square test for homogeneity appropriate? How else could you determine the expected values?

Let's look at an example. Say you suspect that you are interested in the proportion of people from different ethnic backgrounds who are recruited into nurse training. Obviously ethnicity is nominal-level data and you are looking for an association: is nurse training associated with a particular ethnic group? So you want to use a χ^2 test. The hypothesis under test is that there is an association between a particular ethnic group and nurse training. The null hypothesis is of course that there is no association.

The next step after formulating the hypothesis is to record the number of students of each ethnic group entering nurse education. (Your population will probably be defined by a geographic area, see Chapter 3.) In this case let us say that we are interested in the east London area. These data then become the observations. In Table 15.1 there are some hypothetical values. It is important not to convert your data into proportions or percentages.

For simplicity's sake we have used just three ethnic groups and we look at the ethnicity of a first-year cohort of students training to work with adult patients. These data become the observations. The expected values that you calculate are dependent on what the theoretical expectations might be. In this example if there were no association between nurse training and a particular ethnic group, it would be reasonable to expect the ethnic groups to be represented in a manner that reflected the local community.

Table 15.2   Observed and expected frequencies of four ethnic groups in a classroom of student nurses

Frequency	White (UK and EU)	Caribbean	Indian subcontinent	Total (from these groups)
Observed	34	62	28	124
Expected	59.5	41	23.5	124

If we take the east London ethnic make-up to be similar to that of the London Borough of Hackney we should expect 48 per cent to be white, 33 per cent to

> **Expected frequencies:**
> - For males $= 62 \times 0.5 = 31$.
> - For females $= 62 \times 0.5 = 31$.

be Caribbean and 19 per cent to be from the Indian subcontinent. We can now calculate the expected frequencies, by simply multiplying the total number of students by the proportion of each of the classes (white, Caribbean and Indian subcontinent). We can thus produce a table (15.2) that shows both observed and expected frequencies for each category.

Having calculated the expected frequencies, you can perform the χ^2 test as follows:

$$\chi^2 = \sum \frac{(O-E)^2}{E} = \frac{(34-59.5)^2}{59.5} + \frac{(62-41)^2}{41} + \frac{(28-23.5)^2}{23.5}$$

$$\chi^2 = \frac{(-25.5)^2}{59.5} + \frac{(21)^2}{41} + \frac{(4.5)^2}{23.5}$$

$$\chi^2 = \frac{650.25}{59.5} + \frac{441}{41} + \frac{20.25}{23.5}$$

$$\chi^2 = 10.9 + 10.7 + 0.86 = 22.46$$

Thus $\chi^2 = 22.46$. You must now look up this value in the χ^2 distribution tables, but as with all statistical tests you need to know how many degrees of freedom you have. For

> Notice how the values are larger the more the observed value differs from that expected.

the χ^2 test for homogeneity, the degrees of freedom are given by the number of categories -1. In this case there are three categories (white, Caribbean and Indian subcontinent), so there are two degrees of freedom.

The χ^2 distribution table, at $P = 0.05$ with two degrees of freedom, gives a value of 5.99 (Appendix 2). Thus, as our value is much larger than this value we can say that there is a significant difference at $P < 0.05$. In fact our value for χ^2 is greater than the critical value at $P = 0.01$ as well. So we could also say that the difference is significant at $P < 0.01$. We can conclude that there is a significant association between nurse training and ethnic group. There are fewer white (UK and EU) people than expected and more people of Afro-Caribbean origin entering nurse training at this particular site.

Box 15.3

Goodness of fit and chi-square tests

You might be asking yourself what is the difference between the test we used for looking at goodness of fit and those described here? The answer is, very little. The main difference is that in the goodness of fit tests the expected values were calculated using a mathematical model, not real data. As all mathematical models are hypothetical when we use them to produce expected values, we lose more degrees of freedom than if the expected values are calculated using real data.

A specific type of χ^2 exists where the expected categories are all equal. Say for example you were looking for an association based on sex, it would probably be reasonable to suggest that the expected frequencies should be 50 per cent male and 50 per cent female. This type of χ^2 where the expected frequencies are equal is known as the χ^2 test for homogeneity. The calculations for this test are exactly the same as for those described above.

Things to look out for

Yates correction: a correction for a limited number of groups

Sometimes when you have just two categories (say you are looking for an association with a particular sex) you will end up having to use just one degree of freedom. In that case a correction must be applied. This correction is called Yates's correction. Yates's correction involves a slight alteration of the formula for calculating the x^2 statistic. The new formula is:

$$x^2 = \sum \frac{(|O - E| - 0.5)^2}{E}$$

Box 15.4

Practice

Sample the sex of a group of people. Use a x^2 test to see if there is a significant association between a particular sex and the sample.

You will see that on either side of the symbols for *Observed – Expected*, that is, O – E of the numerator (the top part of the fraction), there are vertical lines (|), and that this part of the equation is followed by the instruction to subtract 0.5. The vertical bars either side of the O – E tell us to subtract 0.5 from the result of the sum O – E, *ignoring its sign*. Once this process is complete you process the x^2 test as before.

Take for example the sum:

$$(7 - 12 - 0.5)$$

The answer to this is –5.5. However the answer to the sum:

$$(7 - 12 - 0.5)$$

is 4.5. When using Yates's correction the x^2 values for each calculation use $(O - E|) - 0.5$ as the numerator.

Restrictions on the use of the chi-square

If one of your expected frequencies is less than 5 the x^2 test should not be used. Say, for example, in the example used on p. 168 we had divided the ethnic groups into more precise categories. For example, we could have split the category 'Indian subcontinent' into Bangladeshi, Pakistani, Sikh, Indian Muslim and Indian Hindu. In that case we might find that our categories had expected frequencies of less than 5. As this example demonstrates, one way round the problem is to amalgamate categories (as we did to form 'Indian subcontinent'). The problem with this approach, however, is that the aggregated categories may lose their meaning. It would be very easy to argue that our category 'Indian subcontinent' is so diverse that it is not much use.

If you can't sensibly amalgamate categories, and you have expected frequencies that are less than 5, your only course of action is to use a different test. Options available to you are to use a G test or a Fisher's exact test (Sokal and Rohlf 1996).

Independence

When you use a χ^2 test each datum point must be independent of the others. For example, if you were looking at the use of clinics by different ethnic groups, you would need to exclude return visits by the same individuals. Similarly you need to make sure that the categories are exclusive. There should be no way that an individual could fall into more than one category.

Chi-square test for association: two-way

There are instances when we are interested in more than one nominal scale variable at the same time. For example, we may be interested in whether or not exposure to HIV is associated with particular geographic areas. Here there are two nominal-level variables, exposure to HIV and geographic area. In these instances we need to use a two-way χ^2 test, often called the χ^2 test for association. As with other χ^2 tests the basic formula remains the same:

$$\chi^2 = \sum \frac{(O-E)^2}{E}$$

The difference between the χ^2 test for association and those tests described so far is how the expected frequencies are calculated. The method of calculating the expected frequencies is best illustrated through an example.

Box 15.5

List three pairs of variables that you think it might be interesting to explore if they are associated.

In the following example we will look at the frequency of cases of multi-drug-resistant (MDR) tuberculosis across three European countries. In this example we have used genuine data with respect to the proportion of MDR cases (http://www.eurotb.org) but hypothetical data with respect to the overall number of TB cases. We will look at three countries,

Table 15.3 A 2 × 3 contingency table showing the incidence of MDR TB in relation to three East European countries

Country	MDR TB cases	Non-MDR TB cases	Total
Croatia	13	299	312
Czech Republic	6	184	190
Lithuania	123	170	293
Total	142	653	795

(A cell — The cell's row total — The cell's column total — The grand total)

Croatia, Czech Republic and Lithuania. We ask the question, is there a significant association between the occurrence of MDR TB and geographic region? The null hypothesis is of course that there is no association and any observed difference is simply caused by chance.

Having established the hypotheses and collected the data, the next step is to prepare what is called a **contingency table**. A contingency table simply sets out the data in a standard tabular form. To produce a contingency table the categories from one of the variables are placed in the first row and those from the other variable in the first column. To each first row and column is also added a space for the totals from each row and each column. (Table 15.3.) This type of table is known as a 2 × 3 contingency table, because we have two column categories and three row categories. If there were just 2 row categories it would be called a 2 × 2 contingency table.

Box 15.6

Using the following data that relate the experience of childbirth to the type of pain relief used, perform a χ^2 test to see if there is an association between the two variables.

| Experience | Choice of pain relief | | |
	Gas and air	Pethidine	Epidural
First birth	66	56	36
Second and subsequent	102	22	12

What problems could there be with this data set with regard to independence?

Table 15.4 Expected values for each cell in Table 15.3

Country	MDR TB cases	Non-MDR TB cases
Croatia	55.7	256.3
Czech Republic	33.9	156.0
Lithuania	52.3	240.7

Table 15.5 Chi-square calculations for each cell in Tables 15.3 and 15.4

Country	MDR TB cases	Non-MDR TB cases
Croatia	32.7	7.1
Czech Republic	23.0	5.0
Lithuania	95.6	20.8

The next step is to calculate the expected values. Before, when we have used χ^2 tests we have already known what the expected values should be. In the examples in the previous section, when looking at ethnicity, we used the frequency of the ethnic groups in the community; when looking at sex we used the approximate global proportions of males and females and when we used χ^2 in goodness of fit tests we used mathematical models. In the case of the χ^2 test for association we use the actual data to predict the expected frequencies.

When we calculate the expected frequencies we need to account for the fact that the data are distributed across both the variable country and the variable occurrence of MDR. We can calculate an expected frequency for each cell by multiplying the total for the cell's row by the total for the cell's column and dividing it by the grand total. For the highlighted cell in Table 15.3 this calculation would be $(312 \times 143)/795 = 56.1$. Therefore the expected value for this cell is 55.7. This process must be repeated for each cell. We have listed the results for our example in Table 15.4.

For each cell we now have to calculate the value given by the formula:

$$\frac{(O-E)^2}{E}$$

Again, the values for our example are displayed in Table 15.5.

Box 15.7

- How many degrees of freedom would you have if the table had been a 2×2 contingency table?
- What do you need to do in such a case? See p. 172 above.

The next step is to add up the all the individual calculations to produce the overall value for χ^2. In this example $\chi^2 = 184$.

Before looking this value up in the χ^2 distribution tables you need to work out how many degrees of freedom you have. For χ^2 tests of association this is given by $(c-1) \times (r-1)$, where r refers to the number of row categories and c refers to the number of column categories. In this example this equation gives us $(2-1) \times (3-1) = 2$ degrees of freedom. The critical value from the χ^2 table at $P=0.01$ is 9.21. Our value is much larger than this. Therefore we can reject the null hypothesis and say that there is a significant association between geographical area and the occurrence of MDR TB. What reasons can you think of that might explain these results?

There are alternatives to using χ^2 tests. One often cited by textbooks is the G test. Indeed, several statisticians consider that G tests are superior to χ^2 tests. However, we have stuck to the traditional approach because you are more likely to come across the χ^2 test and few computer packages support G tests. If you would like to read more about the G test Sokal and Rohlf (1996) provide plenty of detail.

Having read this chapter and completed the exercises, you should be familiar with the following ideas and concepts:

- Testing for associations
- Calculating expected values
- Testing nominal scale variables
- Yates's correction
- Restrictions on the use of the χ^2 test

Exercises

1   For the study on the walk-in clinic (Chapter 5) perform an appropriate test to see if the attendance at the clinic is associated with a particular presentation. (a) What happens to the result if you group together those symptoms strongly associated with sexually transmitted diseases? (b) What explanations do you think there are for the relationship? (c) Is choice of contraceptive related to ethnicity? (d) What explanations do you think there are for the association?

2 Is there an association between ethnic group and gender with respect to attendance at the clinic? What explanations do you think there are for the difference?

3 Sample the eye colour of a group of individuals. Test to see if there is a significant association between eye colour and your sample group. Use a χ^2 test for homogeneity. Is a χ^2 test for homogeneity appropriate? How else could you determine the expected values?

16

Tests for Association (2) Correlation and Regression

Areas of learning covered in this chapter

How do:	I see if two variables show a linear relationship?
What are:	correlation and regression?
How are:	regression and correlation used? How are they related? And how can they be used to make predictions?
What types of:	restrictions are there on the use of regression analysis?

In the previous chapter we looked at tests for association for variables measured on the nominal scale e.g. chi-square (χ^2). In this chapter we look at the test most frequently used to test for association for variables that are measured on the interval and ordinal scales. This means that the way the calculations are made is quite different from the way we calculated nominal data and how we tested for associations between variables.

The main test for association we will look at is called Pearson's correlation. In principle Pearson's correlation should be used with interval ratio scale data. Pearson's correlation can also be used for data gathered on the ordinal scale when the sample size is greater than thirty. When using data gathered on the ordinal scale, if the sample size is less than thirty the Spearman rank correlation should be used (Chapter 14). Pearson's correlation is used to determine the extent to which a change in one variable tends to be associated with a change in another. The correlation techniques we demonstrate will test for linear correlation, that is, are the variables associated along a straight line continuum? Where one variable is associated with another in this way they are said to be *correlated*.

It is perfectly possible to have non-linear correlations and there are statistical procedures to test for them. They are, however, beyond the scope of this book. If you are interested in following this up see Bates and Watts (1988).

A correlation can be either positive or negative. A positive correlation occurs where as the values of one variable increase so do those in the other. For example, there is a correlation between age and the occurrence of breast cancer. As age increases so the incidence of breast cancer increases. Sometimes we may find a decrease in one variable as another variable increases. For example, there is an association between increasing wealth and decreasing incidence of mental health problems. This is known as a negative correlation.

Regression in some respects is as much a descriptive statistic as an inferential one. Regression is a technique whereby the line that best fits the points on the graph is determined. It is appropriate to perform a regression analysis only if you want to predict the value of one variable from another or you think that the parameters of the line have a significant bearing on your study.

Box 16.1

Correlations (I)

Suggest:

- Three positive correlations between two variables.
- Three negative correlations between two variables.
- One non-linear regression.

Correlation

When we perform a correlation we not only ask if there is a correlation but we also want to know how strong the relationship is. The correlation test asks how strong the relationship is and is the correlation greater than could be expected by chance. The correlations shown in Figures 16.1a–b are perfect correlations. By this we mean that *all* the variation in variable 2 can be explained by the variation in variable 1. If the points were much more scattered the correlation would be weaker, until the scatter was such that there was no relationship. This is the case in Figure 16.1c. Scatter can be caused by error or by the fact that there are other factors

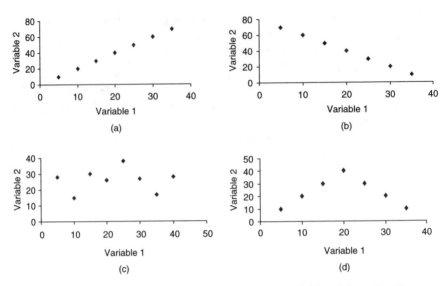

Figure 16.1   Four types of relationship between two variables: (a) positive linear correlation, (b) negative linear correlation, (c) no correlation, (d) non-linear correlation. Note that there are many different types of non-linear correlation

which influence the variation in a particular variable. If we take breast cancer, for example, we know that there are other factors besides age which can influence whether or not an individual suffers from breast cancer. Thus it is unlikely that if we correlated age with breast cancer we would get a perfect correlation. Note that in correlation for every point plotted we have a value from each variable. The values are paired.

Box 16.2

Correlations (II)

Try to find three articles where the idea of correlation is discussed.
    Reflect on these articles and consider how the correlation is used by the authors and whether their conclusions are justified.

The statistic that we calculate to determine the strength of a correlation is called Pearson's correlation coefficient. It is also known as the *product moment correlation*. It has the symbol *r*. To perform Pearson's correlation you must know that both variables approximate (are not significantly different from) the normal distribution (see Chapter 13). In many studies where Pearson's correlation is used the authors do not check for normality.

Table 16.1   Mean pollution levels across ten US cities and the mean peak flow recorded in those cities from women aged twenty five.

Pollution level in 10 US cities ($\mu g/m^3$)	Peak flow mean for females aged 25 (ml/sec)
47	40
9	55
14	50
11	52
23	42
17	44
56	40
110	38
30	44
23	42

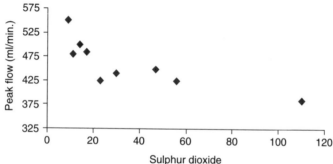

Figure 16.2   Relationship between peak flow and pollution level

How to calculate Pearson's correlation coefficient

First of all you need some data. In general you want a sample with at least thirty pairs. In this example we will use ten, but this is just for simplicity.

Abdo Sadu is a community nurse specialising in respiratory problems and is conducting some research investigating various aspects of lung function and pollution levels. As part of his study he is seeking to establish if there is a relationship between levels of atmospheric sulphur dioxide (SO_2) and peak flow. Sulphur dioxide is an atmospheric pollutant associated with the burning of oil and coal. Peak flow is the maximum instantaneous rate that an individual can expel air out of his lungs.

The first step, as we suggest when dealing with most aspects of statistics, is to plot the data (Figure 16.2). The plot suggests that there is an

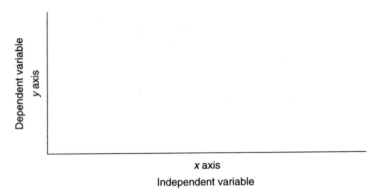

Figure 16.3 Axes of the independent and dependent variables

association (relationship). However, could it just be due to chance, that is, error in the sampling process? The next step would be to test for normality with respect to both the variables, which we discussed in Chapter 13. For the purposes of saving space we will omit this stage.

Now we can get on with calculating r. The procedure is similar to that for the ANOVA test (Chapter 12) in that it involves using the sums of squares. We need to do this for both variables. When we are doing the calculation we will refer to the variables by the letters x and y. Traditionally x is the variable that we plot on the horizontal axis and y is the variable we plot on the vertical axis (Figure 16.3). It is normal to plot the variable on the x axis that you think gives rise to the effect. This variable is sometimes called the independent variable. In correlation, however, it doesn't matter which variable you select to be the x axis. In regression it does!

The calculation you need to perform is to calculate the sums of squares of the cases of the x variable, then the y variable. You then need to calculate the result of multiplying each pair of x and y together. We recommend using a table like Table 16.2. As with most statistics the advantages of using a computer soon become apparent. We used Microsoft Excel to perform the calculations shown in Table 16.2. Using a spreadsheet helps to reduce the number of errors that are made.

Box 16.3

Take samples from a group of people of index and little finger length. Are the measurements significantly correlated?

Table 16.2   Calculation of Pearson's correlation coefficient

Case pair	Pollution level $(\mu g/m^3)$	Peak flow (ml/sec)	x^2	y^2	xy*
1	47	40	2,209	1,600	1,880
2	9	55	81	3,025	495
3	14	50	196	2,500	700
4	11	52	121	2,704	572
5	23	42	529	1,764	966
6	17	44	289	1,936	748
7	56	40	3,136	1,600	2,240
8	110	38	12,100	1,444	4,180
9	30	44	900	1,936	1,320
10	23	42	529	1,764	966
Total (Σ)	340(Σx)	447(Σy)	20,090 (Σx^2)	20,273 (Σy^2)	14,067 (Σxy)

* x and y multiplied together

The next step is to calculate the sum of the xs squared $((\Sigma x)^2)$ and the sum of the ys squared $((\Sigma y)^2)$. These values are 115,600 (340^2) and 199,809 (447^2) respectively.

The next step is to calculate the statistic r, the correlation coefficient. This is calculated according to the formula below. Like most statistical formulas it looks more frightening than it is. If you can add up, divide, subtract and multiply then you can do it.

$$r = \frac{n \times \sum xy - (\sum x \times \sum y)}{\sqrt{\left[n \times \sum x^2 - (\sum x)^2\right]\left[n \times \sum y^2 - (\sum y)^2\right]}}$$

Feeding our values into the equation, we have:

$$r = \frac{10 \times 14,067 - (340 \times 447)}{\sqrt{[10 \times 20,090 - (115,600)][10 \times 20,273 - (199,809)]}}$$

After performing the multiplications inside brackets:

$$r = \frac{140,670 - (151,980)}{\sqrt{[200,900 - (115,600)][202,730 - (199,809)]}}$$

After performing the subtractions (remember to do the subtractions in brackets first):

$$r = \frac{-11{,}310}{\sqrt{[85{,}300][2{,}921]}}$$

Now you can perform the final multiplication to give:

$$r = \frac{-11{,}310}{\sqrt{249{,}161{,}300}}$$

Next, square-root the denominator:

$$r = \frac{-11{,}310}{15{,}784.8}$$

and finally calculate r:

$$r = -0.71$$

The significance of r (that is, is there a statistically significant correlation) just like any other statistic? – can be read from tables that show the critical values of r (see Appendix 2). In a correlation the number of degrees of freedom is given by the sample size minus the number of variables. There are two variables in this case, so we therefore have eight degrees of freedom. So, looking up an r of −0.71 with eight degrees of freedom, we see that the relationship is significant at the $P < 0.05$, but not at the $P < 0.01$, level. The correlation is thus significant but not very strong. It should be noted, however, that this test was a two-tailed test (that is, we did not predict whether the relationship would be positive or negative and would be a more significant relationship if the test was one-tailed). Notice also that the relationship is negative. Thus as x gets bigger y gets smaller.

Some studies report a t value as well as the r value. We will not outline the procedure here except to say that the t value calculated is derived from r and most computer packages will produce both.

Box 16.4

Limitations

- You can't tell that a relationship is 'cause and effect' just because you have a correlation.
- Measurements must be interval or ratio scales.
- Samples must have been taken randomly and be normally distributed.
- You can't use time as a variable on the *x* axis.
- Make sure you plot your data before you do a correlation. The relationship should be linear, although you can transform some types of relationship (see below).

Use correlation when you have samples in excess of thirty. If you have less cases use the Spearman rank correlation.

The coefficient of determination

One very simple add-on to a correlation test is to produce what is called the *coefficient of determination*. This is simply the regression coefficient squared. Notice that when you do this the coefficient of determination (r^2) is always smaller than r (except when $r = 1$). What does this new statistic tell us? It tells us the percentage of the variation in one variable that is explained by the other. In the study described above the coefficient of determination is 0.50. This suggests that for our sample 50 per cent of the variation in peak flow can be attributed to the levels of sulphur dioxide in the atmosphere.

Regression

Regression analysis is a technique used to determine the best position to put a line through a group of points on a scatter graph (Figure 16.4). You will want to know this if you want to show a relationship graphically or express it mathematically. Once a relationship is expressed in this way you can use the relationship to make predictions. What is more, you can use the regression analysis to help express the degree of confidence that you have in a prediction. You may also want to know where a line should be placed if you are interested in having a fundamental

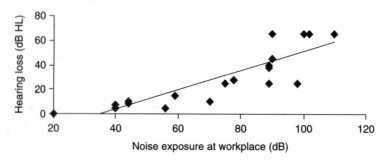

Figure 16.4   Noise exposure and hearing loss

understanding of the nature of the relationship between the variables that are being studied. As with correlation to perform a regression analysis, you need to have measures of two different variables from the same sampling unit. Each single measure of one variable has a pair derived from the other measured variable.

Regression analysis can be used on many types of relationship but here we will confine ourselves to linear regression. Regression analysis as a technique was devised by Pearson as a means to predict intelligence

Box 16.5

Relationships

Think of three relationships between variables that are commonly used in the field of health.
   How were these relationships determined?
   Investigate one of the relationships and explore the nature of the sampling regime.

level and thereby help determine which Jewish immigrants should be admitted to the United Kingdom. Pearson's study was highly flawed but the statistical test he invented is known throughout the world. For an insight into Pearson's study see Gould (1983). As with most analyses in statistics the calculations look much harder than they are. Basic mathematical skills will be sufficient but a computer helps even more.

The line

The line through the points is really a slope, It could be a flat slope or a very steep slope. What regression analysis essentially tries to do is to find a slope where each datum point has an equal influence over where the slope should be. This line is known as the *line of best fit*. Regression analysis can also tell us other useful parameters such as how accurate a prediction would be on the basis of the line of best fit.

What is a slope?

A slope is really a mathematical description of the relationship between two variables. You may have heard the term *gradient* when talking about steep hills. Gradient and slope mean the same thing. In talking about a hill the gradient or slope is a unit of distance along the vertical divided by the amount of distance one would need to travel to descend or climb that distance (Figure 16.5).

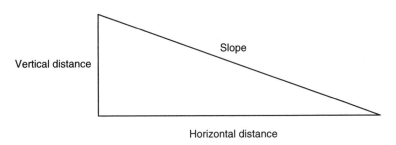

Figure 16.5   Slope

$$Slope = \frac{Vertical \ distance}{Horizontal \ distance}$$

In Figure 16.5 if you moved 30 m along the horizontal in order to descend 5 m the slope would be 5/30 which would equal 0.167. The point about the slope is that it allows you to predict the distance you need to travel in order to descend a certain amount. So if you wanted to go down 110.5 m we could predict the distance you need to travel along the horizontal. We do this by rearranging the equation

$$Slope = \frac{Vertical \text{ distance}}{Horizontal \text{ distance}}$$

to:

$$Horizontal \text{ distance} = \frac{Vertical \text{ distance}}{Slope}$$

so in this case where we want to descend 110.5 m and the slope is 0.167 m we would need to travel 661.7 m along the horizontal. We could also predict the amount of descent given a known distance of travel along the horizontal. To do this the equation would be rearranged to:

$$Vertical \text{ distance} = Horizontal \text{ distance} \times Slope$$

When we carry out regression analysis we are normally interested in being able to predict a value on the vertical axis for a given value on the horizontal axis. You will recall that in graphs we call the vertical axis the y axis and the horizontal axis the x axis, using the letters y and x to mean the vertical (y) and horizontal (x) respectively. Our equation for predicting a value of x from a value of y becomes:

$$y = Slope.x$$
$$(y = x \text{ multiplied by the slope})$$

The equations above tell us the amount we need to move along one axis in relation to the amount we need to move along another. They will actually predict the exact value of say y for a given value of x in only one circumstance, and that is where the starting point is zero (that is, the data pass through what is called the *origin* of the graph, Figure 16.6).

Unfortunately, most data we deal with do not pass through the origin, and so we must adjust our equation accordingly. Think of a relationship between, for example, exercise level (running speed) and oxygen consumption. We would expect oxygen consumption to rise with exercise level (as energy demand increases), but even at a zero level of exercise we would still expect a person to be using oxygen! The relationship between exercise level and oxygen consumption would therefore not pass through the origin. If we tried to predict oxygen consumption from

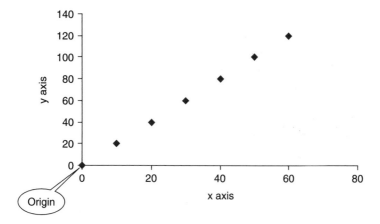

Figure 16.6   Origin of a graph

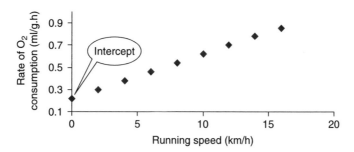

Figure 16.7   Intercept of a graph

exercise level using the equation described above it would not work. It wouldn't work because our y axis (oxygen consumption) would not pass through zero. The point at which the slope would crosses the y axis is known as the *intercept* (Figure 16.7).

To be able to predict a value for oxygen consumption from running speed one would need to start not at zero but at the intercept. Our equation above that related x and y via the slope needs to include the intercept. The new equation is:

$$y = \text{Intercept} + \text{Slope}.x$$

It is normal in statistics to refer to the slope by the letter b and the intercept by the letter a. Thus our equation becomes:

$$y = a + bx$$

Regression analysis is about finding the optimum values for both the slope (*b*) and the intercept (*a*).

Linear regression comes in two forms, Model 1 and Model 2 regression. Model 1 is the option of most researchers, mainly because it is

---

Box 16.6

Investigating slopes

For the relationship you explored in Box 16.5 find the slope (by hand, not by statistics) and express the relationship between the variables in terms of the equation of a straight line.

Try to determine the slope of a flight of stairs, or the slope of a ruler on your desk.

---

available on most computer packages. It is not always the correct choice. We will discuss Model 1 regression with examples and then go on to outline Model 2.

The analysis (Model 1)

Kavita Patel is a dietician working with patients suffering from obesity. She is interested in the weight loss that is associated with calorie-restricted diets. Kavita establishes a study in which 100 obese people are allocated to each of ten different diet groups. Kavita assumes that a reduced calorie diet regime will lead to weight loss but she wants to know, how much to reduce a diet by to produce a certain weight loss.

Each diet is essentially the same but the amount of calories available in each varies, between 2,000 kcal and 1,000 kcal. All Kavita's participants are male and are in the age range forty-five to fifty. All have been referred to Kavita by their GPs and have agreed to take part in the study. Kavita weighed her participants at the beginning of the study and then eight weeks into the diet.

The main function with a regression analysis is to determine the position of the parameters *a* (intercept) and *b* (slope). However, we would also be interested in whether or not the relationship in question is

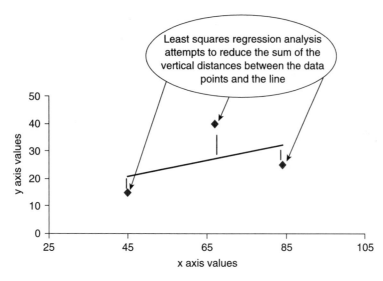

Figure 16.8   Hypothetical slope, showing deviations of data points from the regression line

statistically significant, that is, is the slope significantly different from 0. Therefore Kavita's null hypothesis is that there is no significant linear relationship between the calorific content of a diet regime and weight loss.

The type of regression analysis that we will describe is called the *least squares* method, and what this techniques does is to place a line (mathematically) through points on a scattergram (Figure 16.8) such that the sum of the distance (vertical) between all the points and the line is minimum. The significance of this approach is that it attempts to minimise the error on the *y* axis and assumes that the *x* axis values are measured without error. Unlike correlation, however, the data on the *x* axis do not need to be normally distributed.

Table 16.3 shows the data from Kavita's study. The diet is the independent variable and the weight loss the dependent variable, the assumption being that the weight loss is associated with a particular diet and that the amount of weight loss is dependent on the diet. In regression analysis the *x* axis should always be that which is thought to be the independent variable. In some cases there may not be an independent variable, in which case the *y* variable should be the one that you want to make predictions of from a given value of *x*.

The first step in any regression analysis should be to plot the data (Figure 16.9), in this way you can get a 'feel' for the data and a preliminary idea of what the statistics might show. You can also check for

Table 16.3   Values for weight loss associated with a particular level of calorie intake restricted diet

Diet	Weight loss (kg)
1,000	15.0
1,100	15.0
1,200	5.0
1,300	5.0
1,400	7.0
1,500	8.0
1,600	5.5
1,700	1.0
1,800	10.0
1,900	8.0
2,000	3.0

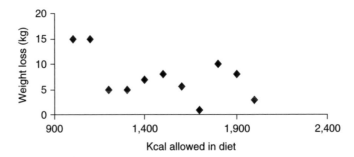

Figure 16.9   Relationship between kilocalories in diet and weight loss

outliers, data points which do not seem to fit the prevailing trend. Care does need to be taken when deciding if a point is an outlier when using small data sets. In a small data set, one could argue, the overall trend cannot be seen and therefore it is inappropriate to call any point an outlier.

Having looked at the data, you need to decide if a linear relationship is reasonable. Do consider other relationships between variables like those described at the start of this chapter. If you decide that linear regression is the best option you can press on to calculate a least squares regression and find values for the slope and the intercept.

The calculation of a least squares regression is quite similar to that for correlation, so you need to find the same parameters (sums of squares for x and y) as you did for correlation. Table 16.4 shows the production of

Table 16.4   Calculation of least squares regression

Case pair	Diet (kcal)(x)	Weight loss (kg) (y)	x^2	y^2	xy
1	1,000	15.0	1,000,000	225.00	15,000
2	1,100	15.0	1,210,000	225.00	16,500
3	1,200	5.0	1,440,000	25.00	6,000
4	1,300	5.0	1,690,000	25.00	6,500
5	1,400	7.0	1,960,000	49.00	9,800
6	1,500	8.0	2,250,000	64.00	12,000
7	1,600	5.5	2,560,000	30.25	8,800
8	1,700	1.0	2,890,000	1.00	1,700
9	1,800	10.0	3,240,000	100.00	18,000
10	1,900	8.0	3,610,000	64.00	15,200
11	2,000	3.0	4,000,000	9.00	6,000
Total (Σ)	16,500	82.5	25,850,000	817.25	115,500
	(Σx)	(Σy)	(Σx^2)	(Σy^2)	(Σxy)

these parameters for Kavita's data. You also need to find the mean of all the x and the y values, and also the square of the sum of the x values $(\Sigma x)^2$. We calculated all the values using an Excel spreadsheet. If you don't have access to a statistical package but do have access to a computer, using a spreadsheet speeds up calculations and reduces errors. For Kavita's data $\bar{x} = 1,500$, $\bar{y} = 7.5$ and $(\Sigma x)^2 = 272,250,000$.

Having calculated the parameters as normal, the next step is to put those parameters into the equations that will enable the final statistics to be produced. The first step is to calculate the value of the slope. As we said previously, in statistics this has the symbol b.

$$b = \frac{n \times \sum xy - \sum x \times \sum y}{n \times \sum x^2 - \left(\sum x\right)^2}$$

Using the values from Kavita's study, this gives us:

$$b = \frac{(11 \times 115,500) - (16,500 \times 82.5)}{(11 \times 25,850,000) - (272,250,000)}$$

$$= \frac{(1,270,500) - (1,361,250)}{(284,350,000) - (272,250,000)}$$

which equals:

$$b = \frac{-90,750}{12,100,000}$$

therefore:

$$b = -0.0075$$

The minus indicates that the slope is negative, that is, as we move up the x axis the slope goes down.

Having calculated b, it is now possible to calculate a, the intercept, by solving the equation for a straight line. If you remember, the equation is: $y = a + bx$, where b and a are the slope and intercept respectively. If we take the mean y values, the mean of the x values and the value for b we have calculated and put them into the equation we have:

$$7.5 = a + -0.0075 \times 1,500$$

We thus have an equation where the only parameter we don't know is a. With a little rearrangement we can get to:

$$a = y - bx$$

Substituting our values produces:

$$a = 7.5 - -0.0075 \times 1,500$$

which equals:

$$a = 7.5 + 11.25$$

and thus:

$$a = 18.75$$

Our final equation for Kavita's data is thus:

$$y = 18.75 - 0.0075x$$

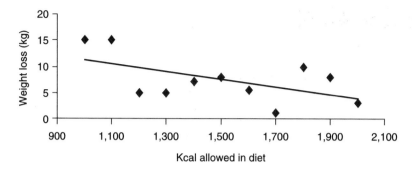

Figure 16.10   Reading a predicition from a regression equation. For a given value of *x* read the predicition from the *y* axis

If you want to make a prediction using the line, take a value of *x* – in the case of Kavita's work a diet of a certain calorific content – and then, using the equation, make a prediction. So for a value of *x* of 1,200, Kavita's equation predicts a weight loss of 9.75 kg.

You could also make a prediction by drawing the line on the original graph. To do this make a prediction for a value of *x* at both extremes of the range of the *x* values. Plot the prediction on the graph and join the two points together with a straight line (Figure 16.10). You can then read from the straight line a prediction for any given value of *x*. But how good is that estimate?

Quality of a prediction

It is important to remember that a regression line is a statistic. Not only that, but normally it is a statistic based on a sample. In Kavita's case the sample is of obese individuals. When we produce a regression line from a sample, just like when we produce a mean from a sample, it is an estimate of where the line would lie for the population as a whole. This means that a prediction will carry error. In fact any prediction will carry with it two types of error, the error caused by the fact we are using a sample and the error caused by the scatter of points around the line.

The 95 per cent confidence limits (Chapter 10) for an individual prediction are given by the equation:

$$CL_{95\%} = y' \pm t \times s_r \sqrt{1 + \frac{1}{n} + \frac{(x' - \bar{x})^2}{\sum x^2 - \frac{(\sum x)^2}{n}}}$$

Box 16.7

Regression

From the data that you collected for the exercise in Box 16.3 calculate a
regression line, using the index finger as the *x* axis.
   Predict the length of an individual's little finger whose index finger is 7 cm.
How accurate is your prediction?

---

where $CL_{95\%}$ is a 95 per cent confidence level. You will have met all the
symbols before except x', y' and s_r. The symbol x' tells us that we are
referring to a single value of x and the y' a single value of y. The confidence limit is of course for the y value predicted by the value of x. The
s_r in the equation is the standard error of the regression line. Just like the
standard error of the mean, discussed in earlier chapters, it is a measure
of how close the estimated value of the slope is to that of the true population. You may remember that s normally denotes some sort of variance and indeed s_r is derived from the residual variance s_r^2. The value of
t used is that from the statistical tables for the distribution of t (see
Appendix 2) for the appropriate degrees of freedom. In regression analysis
with two variables this is given by $n-2$.
   The residual variance s_r^2 is calculated using the equations:

$$S_r^2 = \frac{1}{n-2}\left(\sum y^2 - \frac{(\sum y)^2}{n} - \frac{\left(\sum xy - \frac{\sum x \sum y}{n}\right)^2}{\sum x^2 - \frac{(\sum x)^2}{n}}\right)$$

As with most statistical equations, there is nothing more than the
standard mathematical functions to do here, but it is quite complex
and working by hand you need to take it one step at a time and be
patient. Below we calculate s_r^2 for Kavita's data. Fortunately the only
new parameter we need to calculate is $(\sum y)^2$. The others can come
from Table 16.4 on p. 191. We will show some but, to save space, not
all the steps.

$$S_r^2 = \frac{1}{9} \times \left(817.25 - \frac{6{,}806.25}{11} - \frac{\left(115{,}500 - \frac{16{,}500 \times 82.5}{11}\right)^2}{25{,}850{,}000 - \frac{272{,}250{,}000}{11}}\right)$$

$$S_r^2 = \frac{1}{9} \times \left(817.25 - 618.75 - \frac{(115,500 - 123,750)^2}{1,100,000}\right)$$

$$S_r^2 = \frac{1}{9} \times (817.25 - 618.75 - 61.875) = S_r^2 = 0.111 \times 136.25 =$$
$$S_r^2 = 15.123$$

Thus:

$$S_r = \sqrt{15.123} = 3.88$$

This value is the standard error of the slope, in other words we are saying that we are about 66 per cent confident that the position of the slope of the population is anywhere in the range −0.0075 ± 3.88.

To calculate the confidence limits for a particular estimate we must plug the value we have for the standard error of the slope into equation 1 (below) which was outlined previously:

$$CL_{95\%} = y' \pm t \times s_r \sqrt{1 + \frac{1}{n} + \frac{(x' - \bar{x})^2}{\sum x^2 - \frac{(\sum x)^2}{n}}}$$

In the example below Kavita is interested in a prediction based on an x value of 1,200. From the equation for her regression line this gives her a predicted y value of 9.75:

$$CL_{95\%} = 9.75 \pm t \times 3.88 \sqrt{1 + \frac{1}{n} + \frac{(1,200 - 1,500)^2}{25,850,000 - \frac{272,250,000}{11}}}$$

$$CL_{95\%} = 9.75 \pm t \times 3.88 \sqrt{1 + 0.091 + \frac{90,000}{1,100,000}}$$

$$CL_{95\%} = 9.75 \pm t \times 3.88 \sqrt{1.172}$$
$$CL_{95\%} = 9.75 \pm t \times 3.88 \times 1.08$$

t at $P = 0.05$ (95 per cent confidence) = 2.306, thus the 95 per cent confidence limit for a prediction based on 1,200 kcal is 9.75 kilograms ± 9.67.

Is the relationship between the variables significant?

If you were Kavita you might now be thinking that this is a fairly poor prediction, and you would probably check to see if the regression between the two variables was actually significant. We check this by calculating a t value for the slope. The equation for this is as follows:

$$t = b \times \sqrt{\frac{\sum x^2 - \frac{(\sum x)^2}{n}}{s_r^2}}$$

The values from Kavita's study are as follows:

$$t = -0.0075 \times \sqrt{\frac{25,850,000 - \frac{272,250,000}{11}}{15.123}}$$

$$t = -0.0075 \times \sqrt{\frac{25,850,000 - \frac{272,250,000}{11}}{15.123}}$$

$$t = -0.0075 \times \sqrt{72,736.89} = -0.0075 \times 269.69$$

$$t = 2.022$$

This value can now be looked up in the t distribution tables (ignore the minus sign). The critical value at $P = 0.05$ and eight degrees of freedom is 2.262. As such the calculated value of t is less than the critical value and we can say that the slope of the relationship between the two variables does not significantly differ from zero. Therefore diet type (calorific content) is not a good predictor of weight loss.

Box 16.8

Regression

From the data that you collected for the exercise in Box 16.3 that you have calculated a regression line for, determine if the variables are significantly correlated.

You are probably thinking that we have produced a lot of calculations to reach the conclusion that the variables are not significant. However, we wanted to go through the process of forming an estimation for the parameters of the slope first in order to emphasise that the focus of *bivariate* (two variables) linear regression analysis should be the slope rather than whether there is a relationship. It would be wise, however, if, working without a stats package, you have doubts, to test if there is a relationship before proceeding with a determination of the slope. In practice, when asked to perform a regression analysis, most computer packages will produce all the required statistics, including regression coefficients and coefficients of determination.

Box 16.9

Restrictions on the use of least squares regression

- Use linear regression only when you believe that the relationship between the variables (after transforming if necessary) conforms to a linear-type model.
- The data should be measured on the interval or ratio scales.
- The level of error in the y axis should be constant across the range of y values, i.e the level of scatter should be constant either side of the line across the whole distance of the line. If it isn't, don't use least squares regression analysis. Try the Spearman rank instead.
- Regression makes no assumptions about normality on the x axis, and so can be used in situations where time forms the x axis.
- When quoting the statistics for a regression analysis: quote the equation for the slope; if it is significant and at what level; give a P value and the sample size. Oddly the correlation coefficient (r) has no meaning in regression analysis but is often quoted. If quoting a prediction from a regression equation the error of estimation should always be given.

As well as producing error estimates for the slope it is also possible to do so for the intercept term, b. For the sake of parsimony we will not discuss these here. Details can be found in Sokal and Rohlf (1996). Most statistical packages will produce error statistics for the intercept alongside the other regression statistics.

Model 2 regression

When you are regressing two variables together, whether to use Type 2 regression is a consideration only when you are interested in the functional significance of the slope. This could be the case if you wanted to understand why a certain variable – say, metabolic rate – increases with increasing body mass. Here you want to go beyond description and prediction and towards understanding. The first type of regression we described is perfectly adequate in most situations. In a few cases, however, Type 2 regression is required.

Box 16.10

Model 2 regression

Using the data from the two previous boxes, decide which regression model should best be used to determine the functional significance of the regression line.

The most common situation it is required in is where both the x and the y variables are measured randomly and the level of error in the measurement of both is similar. In Type 1 regression the position of the line takes into account sampling error on the y axis only, and thus if both axes are measured with similar levels of error the line will not be positioned correctly.

You will recall that in her data set Kavita assigned diets to individuals and thus the x axis is not a randomly measured variable. In addition, because she determined the kilocalories within the diet the level of sample error on the x axis is low (although measurement error could be high if the participants didn't adhere to their diets). Kavita was also more concerned with making predictions than with the functional relationship between the variables. Therefore, for Kavita, Type 1 regression is appropriate. An example where you would use Model 2 regression is where you were interested in the size of a particular type of cancerous growth and exposure to radiation. Here both axes are likely to be randomly sampled and to be normally distributed.

Unfortunately most computer programmes do not easily enable the computation of Type 2 regression, and therefore Model 1 regression analysis is sometimes used inappropriately. A quick 'rough-and-ready' method to determine the slope in situations where a Model 2 regression is required is to divide the slope by r, the correlation coefficient. Alternative and more sophisticated methods do exist, for example

Bartlett's three-group method, Kendall's robust line fit, and major axis regression. (Kendall's robust line fit is a non-parametric method.)

Not linear

It is important to remember that linear regression is an approach that assumes your data conform to a linear model (i.e. fall approximately along a straight line). This is why it is important to plot your data before you do anything else.

In many cases your data will not be linear (for instance, bacterial growth over time) and as such, in the first instance, linear regression is not appropriate. Computer stats packages do often have facilities for performing what is known as 'non-linear regression'. However, the use of these techniques and their interpretation is rather complex. In addition, if you do not have access to such packages, then an alternative strategy is required.

Fortunately, for many types of non-linear relationship between variables, it is possible to transform the data so that the relationship between the variables takes on a linear form. Shown in Figure 16.11 is the relationship between metabolic rate and body weight for adult males. Clearly, for these, data linear regression would not be appropriate unless we transformed the data such that they became linear.

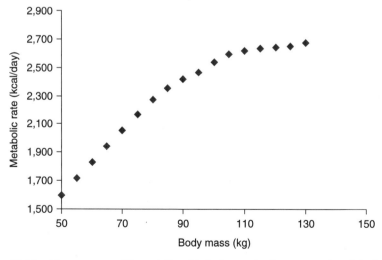

Figure 16.11   Linear curve of the relationship between body mass and metabolic rate

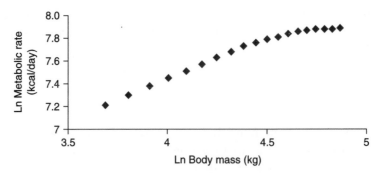

Figure 16.12   Logarithmic curve of the relationship between body mass and metabolic rate

To straighten this type of curve (often called asymptotic) we can take the natural logarithm of both the *x* and the *y* axes. The resulting curve is shown in Figure 16.12. The line is not completely straight but it is suitable for regression analysis based on a linear model. If you perform such an analysis the resulting line will have the formula:

Ln Metabolic rate $= a + b \times$ Ln Body mass.

Other common forms of transformation include logging only one of the axes, the reciprocal transformation (take the reciprocal of the *y* axis) and the Probit transformation. (For information on these see Sokal and Rohlf 1996.)

Multiple regression

Sometimes we are interested in phenomena that may be affected by and correlated with a variety of different variables. For example, in thinking of a person's chance of getting heart disease, we know there are a range of important independent variables such as smoking, the amount of exercise taken and obesity that are correlated with the risk of suffering from a myocardial infarction. The technique we need to use if we want to consider the influence of a variety of independent variables on a dependent variable is called multiple regression. Multiple regression is a common technique but beyond the scope of this book. If you wish to investigate further try Allison (1999).

Having read this chapter and completed the exercises, you should be familiar with the following ideas and concepts:

- Testing for association
- Using correlation
- Using least squares linear regression
- The coefficient of determination
- The correlation coefficient
- The difference between correlation and regression.
- Making predictions using least squares regression
- Determining the accuracy of predictions using least squares
- Model 2 regression
- Transforming non-linear relationships

Exercises

1   For the study on Symphadiol presented in Chapter 5 perform an appropriate test to see if the weight loss of the participant significantly correlates with the height of the participant. (a) Plot the relationship. (b) What explanations do you think there are for this relationship? (c) Is the relationship a strong one? (d) Predict the weight of an individual who is 170 cm tall. (e) What do you think gives rise to the variations around the slope? (f) What is the standard error of the slope you have calculated?

2   Identify three studies from the literature in which least squares regression is used. For each study (a) note the size of the sample; (b) indicate if the restrictions on least squares regression have been adhered to; (c) if the test selection was inappropriate, discuss how you might believe this could change the conclusions.

17

Analysing Data from Systematic Reviews

Areas of learning covered in this chapter

How can   I use statistics to help inform care decisions?
What are   NNTs and L'Abbé plots?
How are   NNTs and L'Abbé plots calculated?

There are many books that look at the research process. Most of them will serve as guides to looking at the quality of published research, and we urge you to use such sources, so as to become a critical reader and user of research. The aim of this chapter is to introduce two statistical procedures that can help you look at published work and decide whether the procedure or practice would benefit your clients or patients. The focus of the chapter is on work that has been published in systematic reviews. The two procedures we will introduce are known as L'Abbé plots and Numbers Needed to Treat (NNT).

We will first note a few important points about using research from other people's studies. The first and possibly the most important principle is that of 'reader beware'. Quite simply, you can't blame the author if it doesn't work for you, or if the study is poor. It is up to you to make a decision on the worth and applicability of the work to your patients or clients. You need to think about things like the sample sizes, the study populations, whether your patients are the same types of patients as those used in the study, was the study randomised, was it a **double-blind study**, does the analysis seem sensible (McQuay and Moore 1997)?

The advantage of using a **systematic review** is that authors should state clearly what quality criteria they used for a study to be included in their review, and of course the review should contain the majority of the available studies published on a particular subject.

Box 17.1

Clinical trials

A clinical trial is where a particular intervention is put under a rigorous test. In these trials some of the participants are given the intervention, whilst others receive no treatment or a placebo. The latter group is the control.

- Review some clinical trials; observe how the outcomes of the trials are expressed.
- What is a placebo, why are they used?
- Can a placebo be an effective treatment?

L'Abbé plots and NNTs help us to give clinical and practical meaning to the numerical data published in clinical studies. Most of these types of data reside in the medical literature. However, as roles within the caring professions change it is important for the basis on which clinical decisions are made to be understood by all health practitioners.

Numbers Needed to Treat

If you read through some reviews or even original papers that discuss new clinical procedures you will notice that quite often the final result is given in terms of risk. In addition the statistical analysis is often focused on if there is a difference between the treatment and control rather than the magnitude of the difference (that is, how well does the treatment work?). Indeed, this goes back to the discussion in Chapter 8 on the difference between statistical and clinical significance.

The 'risks' published are often expressed in terms of a probability and therefore a value from 0 to 1 (see Chapter 9). The risk is the chance of an event such as a disease occurring. If the treatment is beneficial the risk of the event occurring should decrease in relation to the control group. For example, if you treat a group of individuals who have an open wound with an appropriate antibiotic, and another group with a placebo, the

risk of infection should be less in the treatment group. It is important to
remember, however, that in the case of the antibiotic treatment aimed at
'cure' rather than prevention we would expect the number of 'events',
that is, 'cured' patients, to increase in the treatment group.

The NNT statistic gives us a value that suggests how many patients we
would need to treat in order to achieve the desired outcome in one individual. Ideally the NNT should therefore be 1, that is, treat one patient
and obtain one beneficial effect. In real life, however, such is seldom the
case (*Bandolier* 1999).

To illustrate, we will use the following example taken from a systematic review. Moore and Philips (1996) looked at the effectiveness of protein pump inhibitors and histamine antagonists as treatments for reflux
oesophagitis, a condition whereby the stomach contents are regurgi-
tated into the oesophagus. In most people this condition is rare. In some
it can become frequent and the acid nature of the stomach contents can
cause considerable injury to the oesophagus. One of the studies Moore
and Philips looked at involved the use of the drug omeprazole, a protein
pump inhibitor. We will follow their results.

Box 17.2

Prophylaxis and treatment

In the case of a prophylactic intervention, it is appropriate to talk in terms of
the intervention reducing the risk of the pathology occurring. In the case of
treatments of an existing condition it is less appropriate, and here we talk
about the risk of an event.

In the omeprazole review the study group was divided into three, a
control group and two experimental groups each of which received a
different dose of the drug. The experimenters found that they achieved
the same outcomes irrespective of the dose and so NNT was calculated
by combining both experimental groups. In total, forty six patients
were assigned to the control group and 184 to the treatment group.
Of the control (placebo) group seven showed the desired outcome, that
is, recovery, whilst in the treatment group 134 did. This is all the information we need to calculate the relative and absolute risk as well as
the NNT.

The risk, in this case of the treatment working for the experimental group, is 134/184 = 0.72 and in the case of the control is 7/46 = 0.15. This tells us that of 100 people on the treatment seventy two will have a positive outcome, whilst of 100 people in the placebo group only fifteen will have a positive outcome. Any comparison of treatments will need to take into account the fact that some of the 'treatment effect' may be in fact 'placebo' in nature. The **relative event risk** is the likelihood of the event, with the treatment divided by that with the placebo, 0.72/0.15 = 4.8. This suggests that a positive outcome is 4.8 times more likely with the treatment than with the placebo.

The only problem with relative risk is that if the control effect is small and the treatment effect is also small, but bigger than the control, the relative event risk can also be high. Therefore the clinical impact can be overstated.

The alternative, if one is to present data in the form of risks, is to present the absolute differences between treatment groups and control groups. This is known as the **absolute risk reduction** (ARR). In the case of our example it would be 0.72 − 0.15 = 0.57. This figure represents the difference in the chance of the event between the two groups. It tells us how much of the overall increase in the chance of a positive outcome for patients in the treatment group can be put down to the treatment. The absolute risk thus tells us more about the clinical impact of the treatment. However, it isn't easy to link directly to a clinical situation. Numbers Needed to Treat is a method that converts these risk values into a figure that practitioners can relate to (*Bandolier* 1999).

Systematic reviews tend to give the ARR provided with absolute risk reduction. The NNT is easy to calculate, as it is the reciprocal of the ARR:

$$NNT = \frac{1}{ARR}$$

For our example:

$$NNT = \frac{1}{0.58} = 1.72$$

This means that, for every 1.72 patients treated, one will show a positive outcome.

Box 17.3

Positive outcome

We use the term 'positive outcome'. In a trial involving a prophylactic treatment the positive outcome will probably be no occurrence of the pathology. If you keep to this terminology there is no need to rearrange the equation to take into account different approaches to care.

If ARR is not given then NNT can be calculated from the basic clinical trial data, that is, the data that give the sample sizes and outcomes from the trials. Given these data, NNTs can be calculated thus:

$$ NNT = \frac{1}{(Pos_t/Tot_t) - (Pos_c/Tot_c)} $$

where Pos_t is the number of patients with a positive outcome in the treatment group, Tot_t is the total number of patients in treatment group, Pos_c is the number of patients with a positive outcome in the control group and Tot_c is the total number of patients in the control group. In our example the values are:

$$ NNT = \frac{1}{(134/184) - (7/46)} = 1.72 $$

It is possible to compute confidence limits for NNTs. The confidence limit tells you where the 'true' population NNT lies (see Chapter 10). The confidence limits (95 per cent) are given by the following equation (Cook and Sackett 1995):

$$ NNT \pm [1.96 \times \sqrt{(((Pos_t/Tot_t) \times (1 - (Pos_t/Tot_t))/Tot_t) + ((Pos_c/Tot_c) \times (1 - (Pos_c/Tot_c))/Tot_c)))}] $$

Whilst this equation may seem complex there is less to it than at first sight. Remember, do the calculations in the brackets first. Many of the calculations you know the answer to, because you will have had to do them to produce an NNT. We will calculate the 95 per cent confidence level for the example below.

$$NNT \pm [1.96$$
$$\times \sqrt{(((134/184_t) \times (1 - (134/184))/184) + ((7/46) \times (1 - (7/46))/46))]}$$
$$= NNT \pm [1.96 \times \sqrt{((0.73 \times (1 - 0.73)/184) + (0.15 \times (1 - 0.15)/46))]}$$
$$= NNT \pm [1.96 \times \sqrt{((0.73 \times 0.27/184) + (0.15 \times 0.85/46))]}$$
$$= NNT \pm [1.96 \times \sqrt{((0.73 \times 0.00146) + (0.15 \times 0.0184))]}$$
$$= NNT \pm [1.96 \times \sqrt{((0.73 \times 0.00146) + (0.15 \times 0.0184))]}$$
$$= NNT \pm [1.96 \times \sqrt{0.0038}]$$
$$= NNT \pm [1.96 \times 0.062]$$
$$= NNT \pm 0.12$$

Thus the 95 per cent confidence limits are $1.85 - 1.61$. This means we are 95 per cent confident that the NNT for the population (that is, the true NNT) lies somewhere between these two boundaries.

Numbers Needed to Treat can be calculated for all the studies on a particular intervention, or therapy. They can also be formulated for the range of potential treatments available. The NNTs can then be used to help select the best option. It should not be forgotten that choice of treatment depends on a range of factors, such as cost, patient preference and carer experience, skill and judgement (*Bandolier* 1999).

We can also use the same process as outlined above to look at side effects. In this case, we calculate a Number Needed to Harm (NNH). This value indicates how many patients 'need' to be treated before one adverse response is observed. In general, however, one needs to search wider for reports of adverse reactions, although a good starting point is to look at the number of individuals withdrawn from clinical trials for intervention-related reasons (Cook and Sackett 1995).

L'Abbé plots

L'Abbé plots allow a simple graphical representation of the data from clinical trials. They involve taking the data from systematic reviews and plotting them in a way which makes it relatively easy to draw conclusions about the best option, or at least to get a handle on the range of variation within a set of clinical trials (L'Abbé, Detsky and O'Rourke 1987).

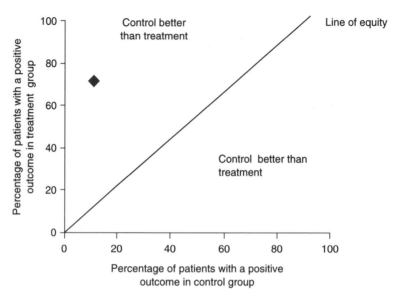

Figure 17.1   Modified L'Abbé plot, showing the line of equity and point for a single clinical trial with the drug omeprazole, used to treat reflux oesophagitis

In a L'Abbé the data from each single clinical trial form one datum point. The percentage of patients who show a positive outcome with the control form the *x* axis and the percentage of patients who show a positive outcome with the treatment form the *y* axis. A point is plotted where the measure for the control and treatment meet. A line can be drawn at 45° across the graph (Figure 17.1). This represents equity, that is, no difference between control and treatment. Trials that fall above the line of unity represent trials where benefit over and above the control treatment was shown, whilst those that fall below the line indicate that the control was better than the treatment (*Bandolier* 1999).

We have modified the L'Abbé plot such that we show the percentage of patients with a positive outcome rather than 'those that improved with treatment' as used in the original L'Abbé plot. The use of this latter term forces the positions of the points of the graph to reverse when cases using prophylaxis are considered. The point shown on the graph is that for the example based on the use of omeprazole that we have discussed above. When many such points are plotted it allows the level of variability within clinical trials of a specific treatment to be seen, and its overall efficacy can be considered. Similar plots for alternative treatments aid in the decision as to which treatment to adopt.

Having read this chapter and completed the exercise, you should be familiar with the following ideas and concepts:

- Risk, and evaluating treatments
- Numbers Needed to Treat (NNT)
- Numbers Needed to Harm (NNH)
- L'Abbé plots
- How the type of intervention, (prophylaxis or treatment) may influence the NNT score
- How to use NNTs and L'Abbé plots to help determine appropriate care plans and treatments

Exercise

Find a systematic review (or several single clinical trials) of an intervention you are interested in, calculate an NNT for each study discussed in the review and produce a L'Abbé plot. (a) Do you think the intervention is effective? (b) In what circumstances is it not appropriate?

18

Choosing Test Statistics

Choosing the correct statistic is sometimes a hard task. The important thing is to think about and decide on the statistics that you will use before you start the study. It is a good idea to write down some hypothetical data for your study and see how they fit into your proposed statistical test. The flow chart is designed to help you select an appropriate test. The chart only covers statistics covered in this text. They are not exhaustive and once you have made a choice make sure to read about the test. Figure 18.1 applies only to the inferential statistics mentioned in this book. Do remember that this book is designed only as an introduction and the statistics described do not represent all those available. If you design a study but cannot decide on an appropriate statistical analysis, speak to someone more knowledgeable before starting.

To choose a statistical test you must consider the scale your data have been collected on. You need to decide:

- What phenomena you are studying.
- How your data are distributed.
- The number of groups (treatments) or sets of data that will be involved in the test.
- Lastly you need to consider any additional restrictions on the test, for example sample size.

We have included a brief summary for descriptive statistics at the end of Chapter 6. If your studying involves using data from systematic reviews Chapter 17 will be of use.

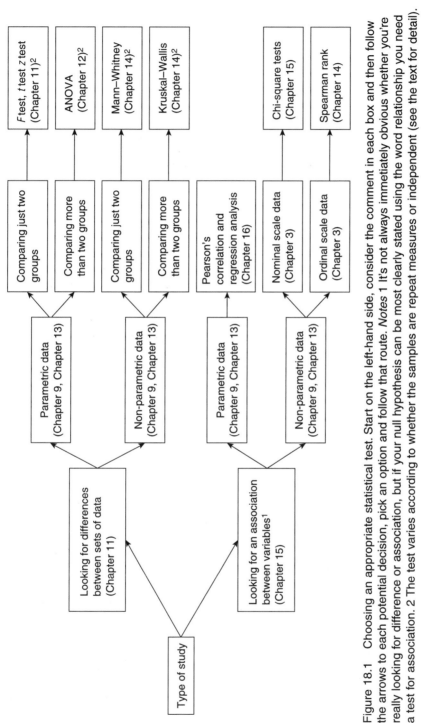

Figure 18.1   Choosing an appropriate statistical test. Start on the left-hand side, consider the comment in each box and then follow the arrows to each potential decision, pick an option and follow that route. *Notes* 1 It's not always immetiately obvious whether you're really looking for difference or association, but if your null hypothesis can be most clearly stated using the word relationship you need a test for association. 2 The test varies according to whether the samples are repeat measures or independent (see the text for detail).

Appendix 1 A guide to Analysing Statistics Critically

This section is intended as a guide to the critical analyses of the statistical components of research, not as a guide to overall research critique.

We suggest that you practise evaluating research. To do so, choose some quantitative research reports on a topic that interests you and work through them, using this guide. Discuss your conclusions with your colleagues.

Population and sample

The very first thing we look at is always whether or not the sample is representative of the population. So you need to look at the size of the sample in relation to the extent of the variation in the phenomena being measured. You need to look to see how the sample was drawn from the population. (Was it random?) Look and think about bias. If information is not given about how the sample was collected, treat the report sceptically. If the data are normally distributed, what size are the standard errors? If these aren't given, calculate them from the standard deviation and the sample size. Always treat studies with small sample sizes with suspicion, as it is unlikely the sample was representative of the wider population.

Co-variables and hypotheses

Do the statistical tests applied actually test what the researchers say they want to test? A well and clearly stated hypothesis should facilitate the correct use of statistics. The most common error to look for is the use of a one-tailed instead of a two-tailed test. The other most frequent mistake is failure to take into account a co-variable or extraneous variables. A similar problem can also stem from design when subjects are not truly randomly distributed among treatment groups (again likely to be a problem with small data sets) or if groups have not been matched properly (again likely to be a problem with small data sets).

Data description and presentation

Have appropriate summaries of the data been provided, including measures of central tendency and dispersion (Chapter 6)? Do the types of measure provided match the type of data recorded? Are the data clearly presented, using suitable tables, graphs and figures (Chapter 7)? What do the descriptions tell you about the data? Can you get a feel for what the data look like? For example, can you tell how the data are distributed?

Choice of statistical analysis

Does the choice of statistical test suit the data under investigation? Is the test suitable for:

- The number of treatments or groups?
- The number of variables?
- The measurement scale(s) used to collect the data?

Has the choice of statistical test been justified? If parametric tests have been used, have the authors tested to see if the data are normally distributed (Chapter 9)? If non-parametric alternatives have been used, are they suitable? Have the appropriate corrections been made (Chapter 14)?

Check that the figures add up, for example that the appropriate number of degrees of freedom has been used and that the outcome of the statistical tests seems to tally with the description of the data.

Are the statistical tests appropriate to the hypothesis being tested. If a one-tailed test is used is it justified?

Discussion

Has the correct hypothesis been rejected/accepted? Are the statistics integrated into the discussion and used with due caution and with regard to the determined statistical significance level? Do the researchers keep their discussion within the boundaries of their sample and population? It is quite common for researchers to extrapolate their findings beyond the original population. If the null hypothesis is not rejected, be suspicious of any reasons that are put forward to suggest why the hypothesis was not confirmed. A perfectly well designed study should not allow room for justification as to why the hypothesis may still hold true if it was rejected. We have to acknowledge that we do not live in a perfect world, but nevertheless reasons should be well justified and not anticipated before the onset of the study.

Appendix 2 Statistical Tables

Table 1 Percentage points of the F distribution, 0.05 level of significance. $v1$, degrees of freedom of sample with larger variance; $v2$, the degrees of freedom of the sample with the smaller variance

v2 \ v1	1	2	3	4	5	6	7	8	9	10	12	24	120	Infinity
1	161.4	199.5	215.7	224.6	230.2	234.0	236.8	238.9	240.5	241.9	243.9	249.1	253.3	254.3
2	18.51	19.00	19.16	19.25	19.30	19.33	19.35	19.37	19.38	19.40	19.41	19.45	19.49	19.5
3	10.13	9.55	9.28	9.12	9.01	8.94	8.89	8.85	8.81	8.79	8.74	8.64	8.55	8.53
4	7.71	6.94	6.59	6.39	6.26	6.16	6.09	6.04	6.00	5.96	5.91	5.77	5.66	5.63
5	6.61	5.79	5.41	5.19	5.05	4.95	4.88	4.82	4.77	4.74	4.68	4.53	4.40	4.36
6	5.99	5.14	4.76	4.53	4.39	4.28	4.21	4.15	4.10	4.06	4.00	3.84	3.70	3.67
7	5.59	4.74	4.35	4.12	3.97	3.87	3.79	3.73	3.68	3.64	3.57	3.41	3.27	3.23
8	5.32	4.46	4.07	3.84	3.69	3.58	3.50	3.44	3.39	3.35	3.28	3.12	2.97	2.93
9	5.12	4.26	3.86	3.63	3.48	3.37	3.29	3.23	3.18	3.14	3.07	2.90	2.75	2.71
10	4.96	4.10	3.71	3.48	3.33	3.22	3.14	3.07	3.02	2.98	2.91	2.74	2.58	2.54
11	4.84	3.98	3.59	3.36	3.20	3.09	3.01	2.95	2.90	2.85	2.79	2.61	2.45	2.40
12	4.75	3.89	3.49	3.26	3.11	3.00	2.91	2.85	2.80	2.75	2.69	2.51	2.34	2.30
13	4.67	3.81	3.41	3.18	3.03	2.92	2.83	2.77	2.71	2.67	2.60	2.42	2.25	2.21
14	4.60	3.74	3.34	3.11	2.96	2.85	2.76	2.70	2.65	2.6	2.53	2.35	2.18	2.13
15	4.54	3.68	3.29	3.06	2.90	2.79	2.71	2.64	2.59	2.54	2.48	2.29	2.11	2.07
16	4.49	3.63	3.24	3.01	2.85	2.74	2.66	2.59	2.54	2.49	2.42	2.24	2.06	2.01
17	4.45	3.59	3.20	2.96	2.81	2.70	2.61	2.55	2.49	2.45	2.38	2.19	2.01	1.96
18	4.41	3.55	3.16	2.93	2.77	2.66	2.58	2.51	2.46	2.41	2.34	2.15	1.97	1.92
19	4.38	3.52	3.13	2.90	2.74	2.63	2.54	2.48	2.42	2.38	2.31	2.11	1.93	1.88
20	4.35	3.49	3.10	2.87	2.71	2.60	2.51	2.45	2.39	2.35	2.28	2.08	1.90	1.84
21	4.32	3.47	3.07	2.84	2.68	2.57	2.49	2.42	2.37	2.32	2.25	2.05	1.87	1.81
22	4.30	3.44	3.05	2.82	2.66	2.55	2.46	2.40	2.34	2.30	2.23	2.03	1.84	1.78
23	4.28	3.42	3.03	2.80	2.64	2.53	2.44	2.37	2.32	2.27	2.20	2.01	1.81	1.76

(Continued)

Table 1 (Continued)

v2	v1 1	2	3	4	5	6	7	8	9	10	12	24	120	Infinity
24	4.26	3.40	3.01	2.78	2.62	2.51	2.42	2.36	2.30	2.25	2.18	1.98	1.79	1.73
25	4.24	3.39	2.99	2.76	2.60	2.49	2.40	2.34	2.28	2.24	2.16	1.96	1.77	1.71
26	4.23	3.37	2.98	2.74	2.59	2.47	2.39	2.32	2.27	2.22	2.15	1.95	1.75	1.69
27	4.21	3.35	2.96	2.73	2.57	2.46	2.37	2.31	2.25	2.20	2.13	1.93	1.73	1.67
28	4.2	3.34	2.95	2.71	2.56	2.45	2.36	2.29	2.24	2.19	2.12	1.91	1.73	1.65
29	4.18	3.33	2.93	2.70	2.55	2.43	2.35	2.28	2.22	2.18	2.1	1.9	1.70	1.64
30	4.17	3.32	2.92	2.69	2.53	2.42	2.33	2.27	2.21	2.16	2.09	1.89	1.68	1.62
40	4.08	3.23	2.84	2.61	2.45	2.34	2.25	2.18	2.12	2.08	2.00	1.79	1.58	1.51
60	4.00	3.15	2.76	2.53	2.37	2.25	2.17	2.10	2.04	1.99	1.92	1.7	1.47	1.39
120	3.92	3.07	2.68	2.45	2.29	2.17	2.09	2.02	1.96	1.91	1.83	1.61	1.35	1.25
Infinity	3.84	3.00	2.60	2.37	2.21	2.10	2.01	1.94	1.88	1.83	1.75	1.52	1.22	1.00

Table 2 Percentage points of the F distribution, 0.01 level of significance. v1, degrees of freedom of sample with larger variance; v2, the degrees of freedom of the sample with the smaller variance

v2	v1 1	2	3	4	5	6	7	8	9	10	12	24	120	Infinity
1	4052	4999.5	5403	5625	5764	5859	5928	5982	6022	6056	6106	6235	6339	6366
2	98.5	99.00	99.17	99.25	99.30	99.33	99.36	99.37	99.39	99.40	99.42	99.46	99.49	99.5
3	34.12	30.82	29.46	28.71	28.24	27.91	27.67	27.49	27.35	27.23	27.05	26.6	26.22	26.13
4	21.2	18	16.69	15.98	15.52	15.21	14.98	14.8	14.66	14.55	14.37	13.93	13.56	13.46
5	16.26	13.27	12.06	11.39	10.97	10.67	10.46	10.29	10.16	10.05	9.89	9.47	9.11	9.02
6	13.75	10.92	9.78	9.15	8.75	8.47	8.26	8.1	7.98	7.87	7.72	7.31	6.97	6.88
7	12.25	9.55	8.45	7.85	7.46	7.19	6.99	6.840	6.72	6.62	6.47	6.07	5.74	5.65
8	11.26	8.65	7.59	7.01	6.63	6.37	6.18	6.03	5.91	5.81	5.67	5.28	4.95	4.86
9	10.56	8.02	6.99	6.42	6.06	5.8	5.61	5.47	5.35	5.26	5.11	4.73	4.40	4.31
10	10.04	7.56	6.55	5.99	5.64	5.39	5.2	5.06	4.94	4.85	4.71	4.33	4.00	3.91
11	9.65	7.21	6.22	5.67	5.32	5.07	4.89	4.74	4.63	4.54	4.40	4.02	3.69	3.6
12	9.33	6.93	5.95	5.41	5.06	4.82	4.64	4.5	4.39	4.30	4.16	3.78	3.45	3.36
13	9.07	6.7	5.74	5.21	4.86	4.62	4.44	4.3	4.19	4.10	3.96	3.59	3.25	3.17
14	8.86	6.51	5.56	5.04	4.69	4.46	4.28	4.14	4.03	3.94	3.8	3.43	3.09	3.00
15	8.68	6.36	5.42	4.89	4.56	4.32	4.14	4.00	3.89	3.80	3.67	3.29	2.96	2.87
16	8.53	6.23	5.29	4.77	4.44	4.2	4.03	3.89	3.78	3.69	3.55	3.18	2.84	2.75
17	8.4	6.11	5.18	4.67	4.34	4.10	3.93	3.79	3.68	3.59	3.46	3.08	2.75	2.65
18	8.29	6.01	5.09	4.58	4.25	4.01	3.84	3.71	3.6	3.51	3.37	3.00	2.66	2.57
19	8.18	5.93	5.01	4.50	4.17	3.94	3.77	3.63	3.52	3.43	3.30	2.92	2.58	2.49
20	8.1	5.85	4.94	4.43	4.1	3.87	3.7	3.56	3.46	3.37	3.23	2.86	2.52	2.42
21	8.02	5.78	4.87	4.37	4.04	3.81	3.64	3.51	3.4	3.31	3.17	2.80	2.46	2.36
22	7.95	5.72	4.82	4.31	3.99	3.76	3.59	3.45	3.35	3.26	3.12	2.75	2.40	2.31
23	7.88	5.68	4.76	4.26	3.94	3.71	3.54	3.41	3.3	3.21	3.07	2.70	2.35	2.26

(Continued)

Table 2 (Continued)

v2 \ v1	1	2	3	4	5	6	7	8	9	10	12	24	120	Infinity
24	7.82	5.61	4.72	4.22	3.9	3.67	3.5	3.36	3.26	3.17	3.03	2.66	2.31	2.21
25	7.77	5.57	4.68	4.18	3.85	3.63	3.46	3.32	3.22	3.13	2.99	2.62	2.27	2.17
26	7.72	5.53	4.64	4.14	3.82	3.59	3.42	3.29	3.18	3.09	2.96	2.58	2.23	2.13
27	7.68	5.49	4.6	4.11	3.78	3.56	3.39	3.26	3.15	3.06	2.93	2.55	2.2	2.1
28	7.64	5.45	4.57	4.07	3.75	3.53	3.36	3.23	3.12	3.03	2.90	2.52	2.17	2.06
29	7.6	5.42	4.54	4.04	3.73	3.5	3.33	3.2	3.09	3.00	2.87	2.49	2.14	2.03
30	7.56	5.39	4.51	4.02	3.7	3.47	3.3	3.17	3.07	2.98	2.84	2.47	2.11	2.01
40	7.31	5.18	4.31	3.83	3.51	3.29	3.12	2.99	2.89	2.8	2.66	2.29	1.92	1.8
60	7.08	4.98	4.13	3.65	3.34	3.12	2.95	2.82	2.72	2.63	2.50	2.12	1.73	1.6
120	6.85	4.79	3.95	3.48	3.17	2.96	2.79	2.66	2.56	2.47	2.34	1.95	1.53	1.38
infinity	6.63	4.61	3.78	3.32	3.02	2.80	2.64	2.51	2.41	2.32	2.18	1.79	1.32	1

Table 3   t distribution

Significance	0.05	0.01	0.001
d.f			
1	12.71	63.66	636.62
2	4.30	9.92	31.60
3	3.18	5.84	12.92
4	2.77	4.60	8.61
5	2.57	4.03	6.87
6	2.45	3.71	5.96
7	2.36	3.50	5.41
8	2.31	3.35	5.04
9	2.26	3.25	4.78
10	2.23	3.17	4.59
11	2.20	3.11	4.44
12	2.18	3.06	4.32
13	2.16	3.01	4.22
14	2.14	2.98	4.14
15	2.13	2.95	4.07
16	2.12	2.92	4.02
17	2.11	2.90	3.96
18	2.10	2.88	3.92
20	2.09	2.84	3.85
22	2.07	2.82	3.8
26	2.06	2.78	3.7
28	2.05	2.76	3.67
30	2.04	2.75	3.64
40	2.02	2.7	3.55
60	2.00	2.66	3.46
120	1.98	2.62	3.73
Infinity	1.96	2.58	3.29

Significance levels are for two-tailed tests; for one-tailed test divide significance level by 2.

Table 4   Chi-square (χ^2)distribution

d.f	Significance level	
	$P = 0.05$	$P = 0.01$
1	3.84	6.63
2	5.99	9.21
3	7.81	11.34
4	9.49	13.28
5	11.07	15.09
6	12.59	16.81
7	14.07	18.48
8	15.51	20.09
9	16.92	21.67
10	18.31	23.21
11	19.68	24.72
12	21.03	26.22
13	22.36	27.69
14	23.68	29.14
15	25.00	30.58
16	26.30	32.00
17	27.59	33.41
18	28.87	34.81
19	30.14	36.19
20	31.41	37.57
25	37.65	44.31
30	43.77	50.89
40	55.76	63.69
50	67.50	76.15
60	79.08	88.38
80	101.88	112.33
100	124.34	135.81

Table 5   Correlation Coefficients (r) for one-tailed test (double the significance level for two-tailed test)

d.f	Significance level	
	P = 0.05	P = 0.01
3	0.805	0.934
4	0.729	0.882
5	0.669	0.833
6	0.621	0.789
7	0.582	0.750
8	0.549	0.716
9	0.521	0.685
10	0.497	0.658
11	0.476	0.634
12	0.457	0.612
13	0.441	0.592
14	0.426	0.574
15	0.412	0.558
16	0.400	0.542
17	0.389	0.528
18	0.378	0.515
19	0.369	0.503
20	0.360	0.492
25	0.323	0.445
30	0.296	0.409
40	0.257	0.358
50	0.231	0.322
60	0.211	0.295
80	0.183	0.256
100	0.163	0.230

Table 6   Mann-Witney *U* test values, P = 0.05

									n_2										
n_1	2	3	4	5	6	7	8	9	10	11	12	13	14	15	16	17	18	19	20
2							0	0	0	0	1	1	1	1	1	2	2	2	2
3				0	1	1	2	2	3	3	4	4	5	5	6	6	7	7	8
4			0	1	2	3	4	4	5	6	7	8	9	10	11	11	12	13	13
5		0	1	2	3	5	6	7	8	9	11	12	13	14	15	17	18	19	20
6		1	2	3	5	6	8	10	11	13	14	16	17	19	21	22	24	25	27
7		1	3	5	6	8	10	12	14	16	18	20	22	24	26	28	30	32	34
8	0	2	4	6	8	10	13	15	17	19	22	24	26	29	31	34	36	38	41
9	0	2	4	7	10	12	15	17	20	23	26	28	31	34	37	39	42	45	48
10	0	3	5	8	11	14	17	20	23	26	29	33	36	39	42	45	48	52	55
11	0	3	6	9	13	16	19	23	26	30	33	37	40	44	47	51	55	58	62
12	1	4	7	11	14	18	22	26	29	33	37	41	45	49	53	57	61	65	69
13	1	4	8	12	16	20	24	28	33	37	41	45	50	54	59	63	67	72	76
14	1	5	9	13	17	22	26	31	36	40	45	50	55	59	64	67	74	78	83
15	1	5	10	14	19	24	29	34	39	44	49	54	59	64	70	75	80	85	90
16	1	6	11	15	21	26	31	37	42	47	53	59	64	70	75	81	86	92	98
17	2	6	11	17	22	28	34	39	45	51	57	63	67	75	81	87	93	99	105
18	2	7	12	18	24	30	36	42	48	55	61	67	74	80	86	93	99	106	112
19	2	7	13	19	25	32	38	45	52	58	65	72	78	85	92	99	106	113	119
20	2	8	13	20	27	34	41	48	55	62	69	76	83	90	98	105	112	119	127

Values are for two-tailed test. n_1 and n_2 are the number of cases in each sample.

Table 7 Critical values of *T* for the Wilcoxon test for matched pairs

	Significance level		
n	*P* = 0.05	*P* = 0.025	*P* = 0.01
5	$T \leq 0$		
6	2	0	
7	3	2	0
8	5	3	1
9	8	5	3
10	10	8	5
11	13	10	7
12	17	13	9
13	21	17	12
14	25	21	15
15	30	25	19
16	35	29	23
17	41	34	27
18	47	40	32
19	53	46	37
20	60	52	43
21	67	58	49
22	75	65	55
23	83	73	62
24	91	81	69
25	100	89	76
26	110	98	84
27	119	107	92
28	130	116	101

One-tailed; double the values for two-tailed test.

Appendix 3 Answers to Exercises

In this appendix we provide the answers to some of the questions provided at the end of each of the chapters. We have given answers to those questions where there is a definite answer. In places we have also added a comment to help you understand what we have done to get the answer. We encourage you to practise your statistics by reviewing papers, joining in research and undertaking research of your own.

Chapter 1

No questions with definite answers.

Chapter 2

No questions with definite answers.

Chapter 3

1 (i) (a) Bone density. (b) An individual woman. (c) Women aged between thirty-five and forty-five who were selected and agreed to take part in the study. (d) Women aged between thirty-five and forty-five who were available to take part in the study.

(ii) (a) The incidence of meningitis. (b) Villages. (c) Villages selected
      for the study. (d) Villages in the south-west of England for which
      data are available.

2   (a) Those individuals who could potentially visit the walk-in
      clinic. (b) Those individuals who visit the clinic and elect to fill
      in the questionnaire.

3   Age: interval. Sex: nominal. Number of partners: ordinal. Sexual
      activity: ordinal. Ethnic group: nominal. Barrier choice: nominal.
      Reason not to use barrier: nominal. Presentation: nominal.

4   Sampling error can be defined as the difference between the
      parameters of the sample and those of the population.

Chapter 4

No questions with definite answers.

Chapter 5

No questions with definite answers.

Chapter 6

1 Mean, 2.45; median, 1; mode, 1.0. (a) The median.
2 Mean, 13.53; median, 13.50; mode, 10 and 18. (Note: these data are
   multi-modal.) (a) The mean.
3 For Exercise 1 the quartiles are 1.0, 1.0 and 2.0 respectively for the lower,
   mid and upper quartiles. Standard deviation is 3.70. For Exercise 2, the
   quartiles are 7.25, 13.5 and 20.0 respectively for the lower, mid and
   upper quartiles. Standard deviation is 8.0.

Chapter 7

No questions with definite answers.

Chapter 8

1 (a) That a daily dose of Symphadiol enhances weight loss in clinically obese individuals (males, aged thirty to forty), compared with just using a calorie-controlled diet. (b) Symphadiol significantly increases weight loss over the course of the study in clinically obese males (aged thirty to forty) on a calorie-restricted diet compared with a control group who use a calorie controlled diet alone. (c) There is no difference in weight loss over the course of the study in clinically obese males (aged thirty to forty) on a calorie-restricted diet compared with a control group who use a calorie-controlled diet alone. (d) Weight loss. (e) The treatment group.

2 Likely sources of error are: sampling error, the difference between the sample and the true population; variation in the sampling error between the treatment groups: measurement error, i.e. the accuracy of the measurement tools; the accuracy of the measurement recorders; design error, e.g. how was the level of compliance of the participants with the experimental design maintained; the influence of confounding variables, e.g. height.

Chapter 9

3 (a) H heads, T tails: HHHH, TTTT, HTHH, HHTH, HHHT, HHTT, HTTT, HTHT, THTT, TTHT, TTTH, TTHH, THHH, THTH. (b) The probability of obtaining any one of these outcomes is 0.0714. (c) The probability of obtaining one tail and three heads is 0.2856.

Chapter 10

1 Mean, 179; standard deviation, 12.25; standard error, 3.16; 95 per cent confidence level, 179 ± 6.2. 3 (c) (i) 109, (ii) 88.

Chapter 11

3 The F test and student's t test should be performed. There is no significant difference between the variance of the two samples

($F = 0.51$, $P < 0.05$, d.f. $= 28$). The difference between the control and the test group is not significant ($t = 0.43$, $P > 0.05$, d.f. $= 28$, (one-tailed tests).

6   There is a small (two-point) difference before and after the lectures. Paired t test (two-tailed) indicates that the difference is significant. ($t = 3.83$, $P < 0.01$, d.f. $= 10$.)

Chapter 12

5   There is no significant difference between any of the treatment groups (ANOVA $F_{3,56} = 2.39$, $P > 0.05$). Below the ANOVA table is displayed:

	Sum of squares	d.f.	Mean square	F	Sig.
Between groups	428.133	3	142.711	2.388	0.079
Within groups	3,346.800	56	59.764		
Total	3,774.933	59			

Chapter 13

1   A χ^2 goodness of fit test suggests that the variable age is not significantly different from that predicted by the equation for a normal distribution ($\chi^2 = 31.36$, d.f. $= 38$, $P > 0.05$).

2   The variable number of partners has a clumped distribution. You may be able to transform these data to a normal distribution using a log ($x+1$) transformation.

Chapter 14

1   There is no significant difference between Asian and African participants with respect to the numbers of sexual partners recorded ($U = 29.00$, $n = 18$, $P > 0.05$).

2   There is no significant difference between ethnic groups in relation to the number of sexual partners reported ($\chi^2 = 1.93$, d.f. $= 2$, $n = 18$, $P > 0.05$).

3   There is a significant negative correlation between the number of partners reported and the age of the participant ($r_s = -27$, $n = 40$, $P < 0.05$).

Chapter 15

1   There is no significant difference between the frequencies of the different presentations. However, if those presentations indicative of sexually transmitted disease are combined the difference is significant ($\chi^2 = 12.25$, d.f. $= 10$, $P < 0.05$). The greatest difference between observed and expected values stems from the large number of presentations indicative of STDs.
2   There is no significant difference between the ethnic groups with respect to attendance at the clinic ($\chi^2 = 14.75$, d.f. $= 8$, $P < 0.05$).

Chapter 16

1   There is a significant negative correlation between weight loss and height of the participant ($R = 0.27$, $R^2 = 0.075$, $P < 0.05$). (c) The relationship is weak, as the R^2 is low; just 7.5 per cent of the variation in weight loss is explained by the height of the participant. Clearly there are other factors at work. (d) The slope of the regression line is: weight loss (kg) $= -22.47 + 0.0202 \times$ height (cm). To predict the weight loss of an individual who is 170 cm tall you must put this value into the equation. The answer is 11.86 kg.

Appendix 4 The common symbols and abbreviations used in statistics

$\pm$	Plus or minus
Σ	(upper-case or capital sigma) Sum of (add up the values that follow)
χ	Chi
μ	The arithmetic mean of the **population**
σ	(lower-case or small sigma) The **population** standard deviation
σ^2	The variance of the **population**
$=$	Equals
$+$	Plus
$-$	Minus
$/$	Divide
$>$	Greater than
$<$	Less than
π	(pi) A constant of value 3.142
$\sqrt{}$	Square root
P	Probability
s	Standard deviation of the sample
s^2	Variance
$\bar{x}$	Arithmetic mean
x	A case or a value
d.f.	Degrees of freedom
a	Intercept of a straight line equation
b	Slope of a straight line equation
H_1	Alternative hypothesis
H_0	Null hypothesis
SE	Standard error
SD	Standard deviation
CL	Confidence limits

Glossary

Absolute risk reduction The difference in the chance of an event between the treatment and control groups.

ANOVA stands for analysis of variance, a technique for looking for differences between means from two or more samples.

Association Where the value of one variable is linked to that of another.

Average A parameter that describes the central tendency of a population.

Bar chart A way of representing data categories. Data are organised in a bar vertically on the y axis and their values are shown horizontally on the x axis.

Binomial distribution A mathematical model that describes data whose distribution is determined by events that can occur as either of two categories.

Case A single value or item of data.

Central limit theorem The theory which predicts that the frequency distribution of the means of samples drawn from any population will approach the normal distribution.

Chance An expression of how likely an event is to occur.

Chi-square (χ^2) A statistic commonly used to compare frequencies among nominal-level data.

Coefficient A term used in relation to a number of statistics; coefficients are frequently descriptive statistics.

Confidence limits An expression of the range of values between which the population mean is believed to be found.

Confounding variable A variable that varies in response to a treatment in a similar manner to the variable of interest.

Contingency table A grid-like table used in tests for association between two nominal scale variables.

Continuous variable A variable measured on the interval or ratio scales.

Control group The participants or objects in a study to which no treatment is applied.

Correlated A term used to describe the relationship between two variables where the value of one variable varies predictably in relation to the other.

Correlation A technique to look for association between variables that have been measured on the interval, the ratio or the ordinal scale.

Cronbach alpha reliability coefficient A measure of the internal consistency of a questionnaire.

Data A collection of information normally concerning a particular subject or phenomenon.

Degrees of freedom A number used in statistical calculations, it is based on the sample size and used because we are working on samples, not whole populations.

Dependent variable The values of this variable are dependent on those of another.

Double-blind study One where neither the participants nor the researchers know who is in the control or who is in the treatment groups.

Experimental group The participants or objects in a study to which a treatment is applied.

Extraneous variable A variable that may influence a study, but is not being studied directly.

F test for equality of variance A statistical test to ascertain if samples come from distributions with a similar shape.

Face validity refers to whether or not the content of a questionnaire reflects the subject matter.

Frequency The number of times a particular value is represented in a sample.

Frequency distribution A graphical representation of the numbers of times each potential value actually occurs in a sample.

Frequency histogram A graphical representation of the numbers of times each potential value actually occurs in a sample, where the frequency is recorded as a horizontal bar.

Gausian An alternative name for the normal distribution.

Goodness of fit A statistical test to help evaluate how well an ideal mathematical frequency distribution fits the observed distribution.

Histogram Representation of a frequency distribution in a graph form.

Hypothesis The proposition or prediction that is being tested when using statistics.

Independent A term that means that a measurement of a variable or case is not influenced by the collection of any other data during the same study. Independent is also a term used to describe the predictor variable in regression analysis.

Independent variable The values of this variable are thought to influence the value of other variables (dependent variables) in the study.

Inter-quartile range The range of values between the twenty-fifth and seventy-fifth percentiles.

Interval scale A measurement scale where the points on the scale are separated by exactly the same amount. Interval scales do not have an absolute zero.

Kruskal-Wallis test A non-parametric equivalent of the one-way ANOVA.

Kurtosis One of the measures of the shape (flatness) of frequency distributions.

L'Abbé plot A method of plotting the results from clinical trials.

Linear regression A statistical technique for describing the linear relationship between two variables that are thought to be related.

Mean A measure of central tendency, the sum of all the values divided by the number of values.

Measurement An observation and record of an item of data.

Measurement error The error that is made when measuring the value of a variable phenomenon.

Median The geometric mean; the physical middle value when all the values are lined up in numerical order.

Mode The most common value in a series of values or cases.

Nominal scale A scale of measurement where data are assigned to a category that is given a name; the data cannot be put into a sequence.

Non-parametric test Statistical test which does not rely on the data being distributed in a manner that approximates to a defined mathematical distribution.

Normal distribution A frequency distribution where the mean, median and mode are identical and the mean ± standard deviation encloses 68.26 per cent of all the cases.

Null hypothesis The hypothesis of no difference, the opposite of the hypothesis being tested, normally that there is no difference between the means or frequencies from different samples.

Numbers needed to treat The number of individuals that you need to treat before being able to measure a positive benefit to one individual.

One-tailed test A test where the hypothesised difference is predicted to be in one direction from the mean.

Ordinal scale A scale of measurement where the values imply an order although the magnitude of the difference between values on the scale is not known.

P **value** The numerical expression of probability ranges from 1.0 (certainty) to 0.0 (impossible). Often quoted to indicate significance or otherwise.

Paired *t* test A technique for establishing differences between means of two related samples.

Paradigm A way of thinking shared by a majority see Kuhn (1972).

Parameter The measures which describe the variables of a sample.

Parametric statistics are determined by procedures that assume data are distributed in a particular way and share common features.

Parametric tests Statistical tests that make the assumption that the data are distributed approximately according to a defined mathematical distribution.

Percentage A proportion multiplied by 100.

Percentile When placed in rank order, a percentile represents one percent of a data set. The twenty-fifth percentile will represent the lowest 25 per cent of the sample.

Placebo An object or activity that is almost identical to the experimental treatment except that it has no, or very limited, biological activity, often used to provide the control treatment in clinical trials.

Poisson distribution A type of frequency distribution that describes events that occur rarely.

Population All the individuals or objects that meet your study's requirements and that you could potentially gather information from.

Power The probability of rejecting the null hypothesis when it should be.

Power test A test that predicts the ability of a statistical test to reject the null hypothesis when it is appropriate to do so.

Probability An expression of how likely an event is to occur, expressed as a number from 1.0 (certain) to 0.0 (impossible).

Proportion Ratio of the number of one category of cases to the total number of cases.

Quantitative paradigm A world view that phenomena can be quantified and measured, predicted and variation-controlled for.

Quartile The physical values at the points that divide the data into quarters when all the values are lined up in numerical order.

Questionnaire A research tool that uses a series of questions to elicit responses from the participants.

Random An occurrence of a phenomenon with no predictable order or pattern.

Random sample Each member of the population has an equal chance of being selected.

Ratio scale A measurement scale where the points on the scale are separated by exactly the same amount. Interval scales have an absolute zero.

Regular distribution A distribution where most of the cases share the same value.

Relative event risk The difference between the impact of a treatment on a pathology and that of the placebo.

Reliability coefficient A measure of the reliability of a research tool.

Repeat measures design Tests that investigate difference between samples, where the samples are made up of the same individuals.

Representativeness Refers to how closely what is being measured is to what the researcher actually wants to investigate.

Robust Statistical tests, which if some of their assumptions are broken, nevertheless retain their power.

Sample A sub-set of the population.

Sampling error The difference between the parameters of the population and those of the sample.

Sampling unit The individual or object within a sample from which measurements are taken.

Sign test A simple non-parametric test that looks for differences in two samples.

Significance A statement that suggests the observation being examined is unlikely to have occurred by chance and therefore should be considered 'real' and should be accompanied by a statement rejecting the null hypothesis and with the level of significance (P value).

Skew A measure of how symmetrical a frequency distribution is.

Sphericity A measure used to evaluate equality of variance, when two or more sets of differences between groups of data are being compared.

Standard deviation A measure of the level of deviation from the mean expressed in a standard form.

Standard error A measure of the difference between the sample mean and the population mean.

Standard error of the difference The standard error of a sample of differences between the means of samples drawn from the same population.

Statistically significant A phrase used when the outcome of a statistical test suggests that a result has not been caused by chance.

Student's _t_ test A technique for establishing differences between means of two independent samples.

Survey A research method designed to gather information about a population that can be descriptive, comparative or attitudinal.

Systematic error Error caused by any factors that systematically affect measurement of the variable across the sample. For example, a thermometer that tended not to measure accurately across the whole range of temperatures under study would introduce a systematic error. This type of error is also called _bias_.

Systematic review A review of previously published information where the criteria for information to be entered into the review are clearly stated by the reviewer(s).

Target group The population that will be targeted in the research.

Transformation A technique to change the mathematical form of data so that it is more easily analysed.

Treatment group The participants or objects in a study to which the experimental procedure is applied.

Two-tailed test A test where the hypothesised difference from the mean does not have a specific direction.

Type 1 error Rejecting the null hypothesis when it is true.

Type 2 error Not rejecting the null hypothesis when it should be rejected.

Value A single case or item of data.

Variable A phenomenon or thing that relates to the individuals or objects under study that varies.

Variance A measure of how much variation there is in a set of data.

Wilcoxon test A non-parametric test that is similar to the paired t test.

z score A measure of how many standard deviations an individual case is from the mean.

References and Further Reading

Acklin, M. W., and Bernat, E. (1987) 'Depression, alexithymia, and pain-prone disorder: a Rorschach study'. *Journal of Personality Assessment* 51 (3): 462–79.

Allison, P. D. (1999) *Multiple Regression*. London, Sage.

Bandolier (1999) 'Numbers Needed to Treat', www.jr2.ox.ac.uk/bandolier/band59/NNT1.html

Bates, D. M., and Watts, D. G. (1988) *Nonlinear Regression Analysis and its Application*. Chichester, Wiley.

Behi, R., and Nolan, M. (1995) 'Reliability: consistency and accuracy in measurement'. *British Journal of Nursing* 4 (8): 472–5.

Bhattacharyya, G. B., and Johnson, R. A. (1977) *Statistical Concepts and Methods*. Chichester, Wiley.

Blakie, N. (2003) *Analysing Quantitative Data*. London, Sage.

Brandt, F. (1928) *Thomas Hobbes' Mechanical Conception of Nature*, (trans. Vaughan Maxwell and Annie I. Fausboll). Copenhagen, Levin & Munksgaard.

Burns, R. B. (2000) *Introduction to Research Methods*, (4th edn). London, Sage.

Colyer, H., and Kamath, P. (1999) 'Evidence-based practice: a philosophical and political analysis. Some matters for consideration by professional practitioners'. *Journal of Advanced Nursing* 29 (1): 188–93.

Cook, R. J., and Sackett, D. L. (1995) 'The numbers needed to treat: a clinical useful measure of treatment effect'. *British Medical Journal* 310: 452–4.

Couchman, W., and Dawson, J. (1990) *Nursing and Health Care Research*. London, Scutari Press.

Depoy, E., and Gitlin, L. N. (1993) *Introduction to Research*. St Louis MO, Mosby.

Fowler, J., and Cohen, L. (1990) *Practical Statistics for Field Biology*. Chichester, Wiley.

Gould, S. J. (1983) *Hen's Teeth and Horse's Toes*. New York, Penguin Books.

Hume, D. (1888) in L. A. Selby-Bigg (ed.) *A Treatise on Human Nature*. Oxford, Clarendon Press.

Kerlinger, F. (1986) *Foundations of Behavioral Research*. New York, Holt.

Kerr, A. W., Hall, H. K., and Kozub S. A. (2002) *Doing Statistics with SPSS*. London, Sage.

Kuhn, T. S. (1972) *The Structure of Scientific Revolutions*, (2nd edn). Chicago IL, University of Chicago Press.

L'Abbé, K. A., Detsky, A. S., and O'Rourke, K. (1987) 'Meta-analysis in clinical research'. *Archives of Internal Medicine* 107: 224–33.

Locke, J. (1975) *An Essay Concerning Human Understanding*, (edited by Peter H. Nidditch). Oxford, Clarendon Press.

McNutty, T., and Ferlie, E. (2003) *Re-engineering Health Care: the Complexities of Organisational Transformation*. Milton Keynes, Open University Press.

McQuay, H. J., and Moore, R. A. (1997) 'Using numerical results from systematic reviews in clinical practice'. *Archives of Internal Medicine* 126: 712–20.

Massey, V. H. (1991) *Nursing Research*. Springhouse PA, Springhouse.

Maynard, A. (2003) '"Tribes in need of data?" Business and management'. *Times Higher Education Supplement* May 2003, p. 26. (Ahead of the future: Florence Nightingale's demand for routine data collection in hospitals is still unheeded.)

Moore, R. A., and Philips, C. (1996) 'Reflux oesophagitis: quantificative systematic review of the evidence of the effectiveness of protein pump inhibitors and histamine antagonist', http://ebandolier.com/bandopubs/gordf/gord.html

Nolan, M., and Behi, R. (1995) 'Validity: a concept at the heart of research'. *British Journal of Nursing* 4 (9): 530–3.

Nursing and Midwifery Council (2002) *Code of Professional Conduct for the Nurse, Midwife and Health Visitor*. London, NMC.

Oppenheim, A. N. (1966) *Questionnaire Design and Attitude Measurement*, (2000 edn). London and New York, Continuum.

Oppenheim, A. N. (1992) *Questionnaire Design, Interviewing and Attitude Measurement*. London, Pinter.

Pearson, A., and Vaughan, B. (1986) *Nursing Models for Practice*. London, Heinemann.

Pittet, D., Dharon, S., Touveneau, S., Sacvan, V., and Permeger, T. V. (1999) 'Bacterial contamination at the hands of hospital staff during routine patient care'. *Archives of Internal Medicine* 159: 821–6.

Popper, K. (1957) *The Poverty of Historicism*. London, Routledge.

Popper, K. (1959) *The Logic of Scientific Discovery*, (1990 edn). London, Unwin Hyman.

Popper, K. (1963) *Conjectures and Refutations*. London, Routledge.

Royal College of Nursing (1993) *Ethics Related to Research in Nursing*. London, Scutari Press.

Russell, B. (1919) *Introduction to Mathematical Philosophy*. New York, Macmillan.

Sokal, R. R., and Rohlf, F. J. (1996) *Biometry*, (3rd edn). New York, Freeman.

UKCC (1983) *Nursing Research: the Role of the UKCC*. London, UKCC.

Index